PREVENTING BIRTH DEFECTS

UNDERSTANDING THE IODINE/THYROID HORMONE CONNECTION

By Eugene L Heyden, RN

Impact Health Publishing

Spokane WA, USA

© 2014

Impact Health Publishing
Spokane, WA USA

ISBN: 978-0-9828276-4-2

Printed in the United States of America

~For Sarah ~

Sarah is a single mom and the mother of a patient who I took care of on several occasions. She impressed me so very much. Her child was so severely handicapped that there was no hope that he would turn out to be even close to normal—and little hope of survival. I had the privilege of recovering him after several surgeries performed in an effort to compensate for his physical defects and extend his life. I watched this mother pour out so much love toward someone whom few would want to hold or even be near. She was so very loving and caring. I will never forget this mother as she held and comforted her little child during the toughest of times. And I will never forget that this little one, under different circumstances, might have had a different life, a happy life, with a future not taken away. It is experiences like this that have compelled me to write this book.

Disclaimer: This book is presented solely for informational purposes. The information contained herein should be evaluated for accuracy and validity in the context of opposing data, new information, and the views and recommendations of a qualified health care professional. It should not be substituted for professional judgment and guidance or provide reason to neglect or delay appropriate medical care. The reader and reader only bears the responsibility for any actions taken that could be construed as being a response to the information contained herein. The statements and opinions expressed by the author have not been reviewed or approved by the FDA or by any other authoritative body. This book is offered to the reader to broaden his or her understanding of the issues under consideration and to help identify options that may be suitable for the individual to pursue, on behalf of self or others, under physician approval and direction. The reader is hereby on notice that the education material offered by the websites listed within this book may at some future time be modified or may no longer be provided. The author and publisher offer no guarantees of the accuracy or validity of the quotations incorporated into this presentation or the accuracy or validity of the information presented by the resources that are herein recommended.

~Contents~

~Preface~

*The availability of THs (thyroid hormones) is critical for brain development. A growing body of clinical and experimental evidence indicates that **even slight decreases in serum [blood] levels of THs can have significant consequences on brain development**.* ~Nucera, 2010, emphasis added

<u>All</u> degrees of iodine deficiency . . . affect thyroid function of the mother and the neonate as well as the mental development of the child. **~Delange, 2001, emphasis added**

Iodine deficiency increases neonatal mortality. We emphasize this statement so that iodine deficiency can take its proper place among disorders that kill children. ~Dunn and Delange, 2001, emphasis added

Somehow, I need to get your attention. The quotations above should help. Unfortunately, few, very few have been told the story I am about to tell. It is the story of an essential element that becomes part of an essential hormone, one that *will* determine the destiny of a new little life.

Perhaps you have previously heard of the importance of both iodine and thyroid hormone during pregnancy, but were left with the impression that iodine deficiency is a problem that occurs somewhere else, not in the good ol' USA, and thyroid hormone problems are easily identified and promptly dealt with at the beginning of pregnancy, making both of little concern.

Boy, I wish this were true! Sadly—no, *tragically!*—both notions are incorrect, placing mothers and their babies at great risk.

In the most advanced nation on earth, thousands of lives each year are shattered due to serious birth defects and the occurrence of challenging neurological disabilities. Autism and cerebral palsy serve as examples. Surprisingly, a good portion of the defects and disability we see can easily be prevented by paying close attention to the iodine and thyroid hormone status of ladies who make babies, both before and during pregnancy. If you are a mother-to-be, or just want to be, please make sure someone is addressing your need for iodine supplementation and has screened you carefully for thyroid hormone abnormalities. Soon, you will learn why this is *so* important. Soon you will learn what needs to be done. Correcting problems here—working hand-in-hand with your physician—will, I believe, substantially decrease the risk that your baby will be born with a birth defect, perhaps a serious birth defect, or a challenging disability, perhaps one most devastating.

Now about the book. It will be different. I'll see to that! Although we will have a little fun as we journey together (fun is just too hard to resist), this is a serious book. Here I want to share with you what the scientists and experts are saying about the issues at hand, so you will hear from them many times in the pages of this book. Some of the quotations I use will be a little on the technical side—placed here primarily for the benefit of the physician, one who may find this book an excellent review. But don't worry, should a quotation used be a little difficult for you to understand, the narrative I provide will explain it all. You can get this! You can easily understand what is being said and what steps you should take. Some little someone is counting on you to read this book. Please read it carefully and, by all means, share it with others. And please share this book with your physician, the one you will be relying upon to make all the right moves. Futures are at stake! Perhaps your baby's future is at stake.

> There is mounting evidence that <u>even mild</u> maternal thyroid under-function may be associated with impaired fetal brain development. (Moleti et al., 2008, emphasis added)

> Normal maternal thyroid function during pregnancy is <u>critical</u> for fetal development. **Deficient maternal thyroid hormone levels during pregnancy are associated with impaired neuropsychological development in childhood, premature birth, preeclampsia, and fetal mortality.** (Burnam, 2009, emphasis added)

Now I know I have your attention. Let's continue our journey together.

~Eugene L. Heyden, RN

Behold the gray box!

I love these gray boxes! I use them in all my books. Each gray box I add to the end of a chapter gives me an additional opportunity to discuss with you other things that will contribute significantly to the subject at hand. The gray box will become particularly useful should you wish to study a particular subject in depth. And since there is more to preventing birth defects than iodine and thyroid hormone that will need to receive close attention, I will pack the gray box with good things to know. Please pay close attention to the gray box placed at the end of each chapter. I placed them there just for you.

Introduction

The fetus is particularly vulnerable to damage from iodine deficiency early in pregnancy, and if supplementation begins only at the first prenatal care visit, this critical period may be missed.
~Zimmermann and Delange, 2004

Development of maternal thyroid disorders during early pregnancy can influence the pregnancy outcome and fetal development. Thyroid dysfunction can lead to premature birth, pregnancy-induced hypertension [high blood pressure], increased fetal mortality, and low infant birth weight. **~Wang et al., 2011**

THs [thyroid hormones] exert their effects on growth, development and metabolism of practically every cell and organ. Their primary effects is the translational regulation of target genes. **~Paquette et al., 2011**

The decision to write this book was an easy one for me to make. I thought of you—a mother whose hearts desire is to provide your baby with the best start in life, free of defect and ready to lead a healthy, happy life. And I thought of how easily this could all be taken away. I thought of your unborn baby, an individual who as a right to develop normally, with a future unchallenged by disability. And I thought of the dangers that lie in wait. Given all that is at stake, I had no other choice. I knew I had to write this book . . . just for you.

In this book, I warn of the threat posed by iodine deficiency and by thyroid hormone abnormalities that occur during pregnancy—abnormalities that are surprisingly common, but often go unnoticed or are identified too late. Here, I will speak of things you have never heard before, but, undoubtedly, things that *you*, as a mother, or *you*, as a mother-to-be, need to know. Trust me, Mom, you have some very bad things to prevent. You may know what some of these bad things are.

Perhaps you have a friend or a neighbor who has a child with serious physical or developmental challenges, conditions that will last for a lifetime. Did you know that a thyroid hormone abnormality during gestation may be the cause of such heartache and such devastation? And did you know that something as simple as iodine deficiency may be the cause of the thyroid abnormality that is out to destroy?

You probably thought (if you thought about it at all) that thyroid hormone is what you reach for when you are chronically tired, when your fingernails are brittle, or when your hair is falling out by the handful. It is, but it is so much more! *This* is the hormone that you reach for when you want genetic events to occur . . . correctly, and right on schedule. Surprisingly, there are between **2,000 and 10,000** receptors responsive to thyroid hormone within the nucleus of any given cell, making thyroid hormone intimately involved in initiating and regulating genetic events (Neves et al., 2002). Each stage of fetal development, in fact the entire continuum of fetal development, is a series of genetic events carefully orchestrated by the actions of thyroid hormone (Morreale de Escobar et al., 2004). Clearly, **thyroid hormone *is* the hormone of embryonic and fetal development. It has so many things to do.** Keep all this in mind as we journey together in the pages of this book. Also keep in mind that you really don't want to see what happens when thyroid hormone is in short supply while a new little baby is under construction. *This* is a recipe for disaster! Of course, you won't see the results of this until later. It will all be hidden from view, to be revealed at a later time in the form of a pregnancy loss, in the form of a troubled pregnancy, or in the form of a life that did not turn out as intended. And you may never know why.

Of course, we can always blame genetics for the negative outcomes we see. But the simple fact is, without proper regulation, even good genes can fail to deliver on their promise. Genes need appropriate and timely orchestration during embryonic and fetal development or the results will be unfavorable. In this context, thyroid hormone deficiency *imposed* on the developing embryo/fetus—even occurring during the newborn period and during infancy—can drastically alter the future, or take it away. How tragic is this? All from a simple hormone. All from a simple hormone that is in short supply during gestation and during the critically important developmental period that begins immediately after birth. Conversely, there are problems that may occur when thyroid hormone is in excess (Morreale de Escobar et al., 2004). So attention will need to be directed here, too, should this situation exist.

I know. It seems that I'm starting out kinda negative here. Pregnancy—and beyond—should be a happy time, a time filled with pleasant thoughts and the anticipation of a bright future ahead. I do not want to take any of this away by concentrating on the risks involved in making someone new—but I will, just a little. I do this only to get your attention and to get my message across (and to prompt you to act). When we are finished here (and certain issues have been addressed), I will let you get back to happiness once again. This is an exciting time, the making of a brand new individual. However, by focusing on some of the problems that real people face, perhaps we can move forward with greater confidence, knowing that we can take matters in our own hands and greatly decrease the likelihood that a child who is brought into the word damaged and beyond repair.

Thyroid hormone metabolism 101

I know. You are not accustomed to using medical terms and thinking about the body's inner workings, and when it comes to making babies, the thyroid gland is not that high in the list of the body parts that usually come to mind. But the thyroid is one very important organ, one that _will_ influence the health of the fetus, the health of the newborn, the health of infant and that of the child—actually the entire life of the one **you** will create. It influences everything! You might think that this thyroid business is hard to understand. But this is where I come in. I can make things easy.

So briefly, what is the thyroid gland and what does it do?

The **thyroid gland** is best described as a "butterfly-shaped" organ, and is located at the base of the neck because something important had to go there. It's actually a little factory! And the hormones that it produces are sent forth to become involved in countless physiological activities. The principle hormone created by the thyroid is called **thyroxin**, or **T4** for short. The thyroid uses iodine in the manufacturing process to create a molecule with 4 iodine atoms residing on its surface. The "4" in T4 represents the 4 iodine atoms used in its construction. The thyroid hormone also produces a 3-iodine molecule called **triiodothyronine**, or **T3** for short (thank goodness!). Both T4 and T3 are released by the thyroid gland in regulated amounts, with T4 accounting for roughly 80% of total production of thyroid hormone (Obican et al., 2012). The remainder of thyroid hormone production is T3. Just so you know, when an organ or a cell creates a molecule which is released into the bloodstream in order to influence another organ or a particular cell, the molecule is generally called a **hormone**. The body uses both thyroid hormones, T3 and T4, to stimulate or otherwise regulate a multitude of cellular activities; and, in particular, the body uses T3, the "active" form of thyroid hormone, to orchestrate the genetic events involved in normal growth, development, and day-to-day living. This is why the thyroid status of the mother-to-be is such an important consideration. The one under construction will, for the most part, depend on Mom to provide an adequate supply of thyroid hormone. The embryo/fetus wants little, if any, T3 from the mother; it will want to create (and regulate) this most potent thyroid hormone all by itself and create all the T3 that it needs, on site. *It wants T4, with little demand for maternal T3* (Morreale de Escobar et al., 2004). If T4 is supplied in sufficient amounts by the mother, the fetus will know exactly what to do. It will use this hormone to create the right amount of T3, in the right place and at the right time, in order to perform specific developmental tasks, and will use T3 to activate certain genes and to repress other genes—in a highly regulated and precisely-orchestrated fashion—to produce both normal growth and normal development (this, you want!). The fetus does all this, all on its own, by the genetic instructions built into the cells. Mom just supplies the raw materials. I hope she is up to the task.

Besides the two principle thyroid hormones, T3 and T4, there is another hormone intimately involved. It is called the thyroid stimulating hormone, or **TSH** for short. The TSH is a signaling hormone produced by the pituitary gland, located at the base of the brain. Generally, if the TSH is elevated, the pituitary is trying to stimulate the thyroid gland to produce more thyroid hormone, both T3 and T4. However, if the TSH is it is very low, the thyroid gland is producing too much thyroid hormone and little if any stimulation by the pituitary will occur, such as seen in hyperthyroidism. If an individual is believed to have a normal thyroid status, he or she is referred to as **euthyroid**.

There is one more important term to become familiar with before we continue. The word *hypothyroxinemia* means low blood levels of thyroxin, or T4. It is obvious that the use of bigger words is more fun than simple little easy words; but here, for the sake of simplicity, we will use the abbreviated terms whenever we can: **T4** for *thyroxin*, and **low T4** for *hypothyroxinemia*, okay? Any other big words that we come across, I'll try my best to explain. Even though we will talk a little science here, this material will not be all that difficult to understand.

And the reason you want to pay close attention to what follows, the reason I worked so very hard to bring this information before you, is because so much is at stake.

Now how easy was that? You <u>can</u> learn this stuff! It's not hard at all.

Want to learn more?

That's the spirit! Now, go find a computer and watch the following:

—**Effects of Thyroid Disease Endocrine Disorders**
www.youtube.com/watch?v=ERH76CNWIM8

—**How a Thyroid Gland Can Become Underactive**
www.youtube.com/watch?v=GJQBJz7VuDE

—**Mechanism of Thyroxine Action**
www.youtube.com/watch?v=mRI_oYGzirU

Chapter 1
It's all about you

Pregnant women are particularly vulnerable to iodine deficiency because early pregnancy is characterized by a rapid surge in thyroid hormone production (and iodine requirements). Late pregnancy also stresses maternal iodine stores because of increased renal clearance. **~Lockwood, 2013**

The physiologic changes associated with pregnancy require an increased availability of thyroid hormones by 40% to 100% to meet the needs of mother and fetus. **~Feldt-Rasmussen et al., 2011**

*The availability of THs (thyroid hormones) is critical for brain development. A growing body of clinical and experimental evidence indicates that **even <u>slight</u> decreases in serum [blood] levels of THs can have significant consequences on brain development**.* **~Nucera, 2010, emphasis added**

This story is about you.

Of course, it's all about you, just as it should be—particularly if you are of child-bearing age. You are *so* very important. ***You*** will influence the quality of the next generation. But how did you get to this point? You somehow made your way inside of someone named Mom, and went from one cell to what ended up being trillions upon trillions of cells—complex cells—and by the strategic use of one very important hormone. So let's see how you arrived on the scene.

Let's start with you, the "one-cell" creature you—and at a time when you were so small that you could barely be seen by the naked eye. You started out as one big cell, the biggest cell the human body will ever make. You, in the form of a single cell, were probably created by your mother even before she herself was born! Then, at just the right time in her life you were released and sent on an incredible journey to find another cell, one that wiggles a lot when it gets excited. *This* stage did not last long! You soon became one big fertilized egg. Boy, you have no idea what it will take to develop into that lovely person you will become, the one that will have a tough time finding enough nice words to say about this wonderful and kind author. What you will do next, as you proceed from one cell to around 100 trillion of cells, is nothing short of a miracle.

As you progress beyond the initial stage of existence, you won't waste any time or money downloading the necessary developmental programs—they are already there inside of each cell, but you will need to activate them, and activate them in a precisely controlled fashion. You will use thyroid hormone to activate, as needed, a myriad of timed genetic programs that will make you, cell-by-cell, one of the greatest creatures that has ever set foot on planet earth . . . wearing diapers! Since thyroid hormone, then and now, is intimately involved in the initiation and control of genetic events, and since you are a genetic event—actually, an ongoing genetic event—you will still need this hormone to be in adequate supply (or else!).

Well, that was quick! Now you are here, all grown up, and with a little reading assignment directly in front of you. It wasn't easy, but you seemed to breeze right through this developmental business, out of diapers (we hope) and into moderately seductive attire. Later, if we have the time, we'll go into exacting detail on how the growth and developmental process occurs. But now, of course, you are responding to the urge to "replicate," rather frequently, I might add. With respect to "replication," you will put thyroid hormone to good use here, too. You will need energy to get this whole thing off the ground (if you know what I mean)! Thyroid hormone means energy. It participates in the energy production that occurs within the cell. In addition, you will need thyroid hormone in adequate supply to pass on to the one who will call you home for approximately nine long months. For a good portion of your pregnancy, **you** will be the only source of thyroid hormone for that little someone who will be continuously developing inside (and developing at an incredible rate). Your baby's little thyroid gland will pitch in to help (a little) around mid-gestation, but, overall, he or she will still require your thyroid hormone contribution in order to continue to develop properly (Morreale de Escobar et al., 2004). And during the entire pregnancy, **you** will be your baby's only source of iodine, the element he or she will need in order to manufacture thyroid hormone, too, just like mommy. See, even when there is someone living and developing within, it is still all about you. Will you be able to deliver on the unspoken promise to provide all that is necessary for the one who is counting on you?

But your baby isn't the only one at risk should your thyroid hormone status be inappropriate during your pregnancy, you are at risk, too. Your risk of placental separation and preterm labor is elevated when thyroid hormone is in short supply (Casey et al., 2005; Román et al., 2013). All of this, of course, places both you and your baby in jeopardy. So while it is all about you it is all about your baby, too. You are both in this together. You could lose your baby, you could even lose your life, simply due to an undetected and unresolved thyroid hormone issue (Hall, 2009; Tudosa et al., 2010, Wang et al., 2011). And don't think that fetal loss and maternal loss do not occur in this day and age. They do. So, while I am deeply concerned about your baby, so much so that I wrote a certain little book, you can understand why I am also deeply concerned about you.

> Diagnosing maternal thyroid dysfunction during all states of pregnancy is very important for the outcome for both mother and fetus. (Feldt-Rasmussen et al., 2011)

Miracle on board

The making of a baby is simply amazing—yes the fun part, but especially the developmental part. You are on one *incredible* journey! If you would like to watch a great little video on fetal development, there are many on YouTube to choose from. Start with this one:

—The Miracle of Life
www.youtube.com/watch?v=GZk4hT7ncv0

Have I got an app for you!

I have this great little app installed on my iPad. It includes images covering the various stages of fetal development, week by week, plus so much more. It is produced by Pampers— you're going to be singing the praises of this company several times a day! The app is called *Hello Baby*. It is available from iTunes and Google Play (for android devices). It is a free app, fun, and, may I add, very worthwhile.

Chapter 2
Just as it should be

*Thyroid hormone is necessary for normal brain development. It becomes increasingly clear that the levels of thyroid hormone required at different stages of development are critical. . . . <u>Not only maternal and/or fetal and neonatal hypothyroidism clearly affect brain development</u>, but also <u>**excessive** levels of thyroid hormones may lead to abnormal brain development</u>.* **~Kester et al., 2004, emphasis added**

<u>*Efforts to detect and prevent maternal hypothyroxinemia in early pregnancy appear fully justified*</u>*. Indeed, neurodevelopment defects, including an increased <u>probability of **cerebral palsy**, may be **150 times** more frequent</u> than those resulting from untreated congenital hypothyroidism.* **~Calvo et al., 2002, emphasis added**

Well, the making of a new child is not going to be easy, and it is not going to be quick. It will take at least three trimesters to pull this off. And things won't occur correctly during <u>any</u> trimester without the presence of adequate amounts of the thyroid hormone we call T4. Keep this in mind as we take a brief look at how a normal pregnancy should progress, from start to finish. Unlike other baby books that barely touch on the critical need for thyroid hormone to ensure proper fetal development (or even mention it at all), this will not happen here. Since thyroid hormone will create this new little baby, it should take center stage.

In the beginning

First, the "magic" happens! (We won't go into the details.) Then there is an egg surrounded by a whole lot of new friends. One friend we will call Fred. Well, Fred is just about to lose his identity! **Bam!** There it happened! Fred beat out all the other Freds and is now **gone!** (He was only needed for parts.) He victoriously wiggled his way inside the egg, surprisingly kept everyone else out, and is now in the process of being incorporated into this very large cell. "Good-bye, Fred! You will be missed." Now begins the cell division and cellular differentiation process that will create an entirely new individual, an individual who will eventually need piano lessons. (This is my favorite paragraph; it took me only three weeks to write it.)

The uniting of two cells, however, does not automatically mean a pregnancy will occur. Fertilization normally takes place in the fallopian tube, a passageway leading from the ovary to the uterus. The fertilized egg then will embark on a 3-day journey to find a suitable spot on the inner surface of the uterus to "dig in" and create a connection between itself and Mom. Once this connection occurs, the pregnancy begins. Not surprisingly, all pregnancies begin at the very beginning of the first trimester. There are no exceptions.

The first trimester

The stage of development during which the lack of T4 in the fetus is most detrimental for neurodevelopment is thought to be the first trimester. ~**Sutandar et al., 2007**

There is increasing evidence from epidemiological and experimental data that first trimester maternal thyroid status is **pivotal** *for the outcome of pregnancy and for the neuropsycho-motor development of the child.* ~**Calvo et al., 2002, emphasis added**

How exciting, this first trimester! Mom gets to throw up a lot. And the food cravings can be <u>very</u> entertaining. But there is excitement in the air! Even though someone has the Egyptian flu—they're going to be "Mummy!"—it is an exciting time, nevertheless; a miracle is taking place. (I hear a choir singing.) And, toward the end of the first trimester, the fetus will have fingers and toes later to be counted, arms and legs with little or nothing to do, and a head that is bigger than anything else!—just as it should be.

So much occurs during this first developmental period (and even before). If the thyroid status is inadequate in the mother-to-be, perhaps even the attachment to the uterus will not go as planned. Hypothyroidism, even what is called subclinical hypothyroidism, a form of hypothyroidism that appears mild and of limited consequence, can lead to reproductive failure (Verma et al., 2012). Once the attachment is made, however, in just a few short days we're making a neural tube needing folic acid. Within a few short weeks we're making intestines that will eventually make a lot of entertaining noises, eyelids that open and close, and a liver that actually produces little red blood cells—a job later handed over to the bone marrow. And, before the first trimester comes to a close, boy or girl parts will become quite evident, but discretely hidden from view.

It is in the first trimester that so many genetically programmed events occur—and at a rate that is almost unbelievable—that a healthy thyroid status of the mother at this developmental period has come to be viewed as *"pivotal"* to the outcome of the pregnancy (Calvo et al., 2002). You were never really told this before. You were told to take a prenatal vitamin daily and promptly report any symptom that seems to be out of the ordinary. Chances are, you were not carefully screened to rule out <u>any</u> chance that your thyroid hormone status is abnormal. Yet, this is possibly the most important thing that can be done, medically, during the first trimester. So important is screening, that the following has been written:

> Unless action is taken to test every pregnant woman as early in pregnancy as possible (or even before conception), our society will continue to pay a heavy price in the number of damaged offspring. (Mitchell and Klein, 2004)

And, may I inquire, was there any discussion concerning your iodine status during your first prenatal visit? (You don't have to answer out loud, unless you want to.) There certainly should have been! This is a period when iodine intake should probably be doubled (Stagnaro-Green et al., 2012). Astonishingly, *"it is estimated that only 20% of pregnant women in the United States use iodine-containing supplements."* (Stagnaro-Green et al., 2012) And why is this of such concern? Because iodine influences the amount of T4 Mom can manufacture and transfer to her developing baby, pure and simple . . . and so very important!

Decreases in maternal T4 associated <u>with even mild iodine deficiency</u> may have adverse effects on the cognitive function of offspring, and iodine deficiency remains the leading cause of preventable intellectual disability. (Stagnaro-Green et al., 2012, emphasis added)

This first trimester is *"pivotal"* in so many ways. It is during this period of life that the organizational details of the brain have their beginnings. Stem cells migrate to specific locations, rapidly divide, and begin to develop into structures, neurons, and supportive cells that turn the brain into the most amazing structure on Planet Earth (Kester et al., 2004). This, however, will not go as planned if iodine and/or thyroid hormone is in short supply. **Serious defects in the brain can occur for this and for no other reason!** It may even have defects resembling those found in the brains of individuals who have autism and schizophrenia (Román et al., 2013; Palha and Goodman, 2005). You should be trembling, at least just a little. **There is so much at stake!** Also at stake are other developing structures that can be negatively influenced by thyroid hormone deficiency. The development of the heart occurs very soon after conception and there is evidence that it may become defective if supplies of thyroid hormone are low during the early days of pregnancy (Mayo Clinic, 1998–2014; Nagey, 2002). Unfortunately, by the time a thyroid problem is identified at the first prenatal visit and corrective action has been taken, the damage may have already been done, underscoring the need to effectively address iodine and thyroid hormone issues even before a pregnancy occurs.

In the next chapter we will focus on what can go wrong when iodine and/or thyroid hormone are in short supply during the second trimester, but we should probably finish this chapter first. Before we move on, please remember that the thyroid hormone status of the mother during the first trimester is "*pivotal*" to the outcome of the pregnancy. It doesn't get any simpler than this. Now that the first twelve weeks or so have passed, it is time to begin another trimester. The second trimester awaits. Fasten your seat belt (while you still can). It will be quite a ride.

The second trimester

> *A gradual reduction in FT4 [free T4] concentrations was observed in a high proportion of women over the course of the second trimester . . . despite TSH concentrations remaining consistently within the normal range.* **~Moleti et al., 2009**

> *Thyroid disease if left untreated will continue throughout the entire pregnancy. Thus, screening for thyroid disorders in the second trimester is also important.* **~Yang et al., 2014**

Another exciting time! Mom is getting bigger! People are guessing! Someone is glowing! And a nursery is in the planning stages. Pink or blue, that is the question.

During this period of motherhood, there is a lot going on. Thousands upon thousands of cells are dividing . . . per second! Eyelashes and eyebrows appear from out of nowhere! Nails are growing on fingers and toes, sometimes on extra fingers and toes! The heartbeat can be heard with a stethoscope. Fingerprints, that one day we all hope will not end up on file with the FBI, are being formed. Thyroid hormone is being used, non-stop, to perform some very important tasks, particularly with respect to the neurodevelopment of the fetus. The fetal thyroid gland, hopefully in the right place, will begin production of thyroid hormone, slowly, then in ever-increasing amounts. But don't count on this to be enough to make up for a lack of thyroid hormone delivered by Mom. The fetus still needs, *desperately needs*, maternal T4 to be delivered in adequate amounts, or the outcome may still be compromised.

The role of thyroid hormone during the second trimester is much the same as that during the first trimester. It will be regulating genes and sustaining genetic events so that development occurs normally and at a proper pace. Developing the brain, building on the successes of the first trimester, will be a top priority during the second trimester. Of course, it is a brain that we are really after. And we want a great one! (Like the one I wish I had.) But it won't be a good one, let alone a great one, if Mom is not supplying enough thyroid hormone to meet the demands of the one who is developing inside.

Low thyroid hormone availability, even at this stage of the game (second trimester), may lead to the death of the fetus (Allan et al., 2000; Ozdemir et al., 2013). This, of course, puts an end to that great brain (and the entire bundle of joy) we were hoping for, and there is great sadness throughout the land. All may be lost simply due to thyroid hormone deficiency in the mother, even when thyroid hormone levels are supposedly "normal," such as seen in maternal subclinical hypothyroidism (Ozdemir et al., 2013). Low thyroid hormone availability is not a rare event, many, many babies are lost due to low thyroid availability and other thyroid hormone issues that arise during the second trimester (Allan et al., 2000). If only careful screening for iodine and thyroid hormone insufficiency had been performed before or at the beginning of pregnancy, multitudes of little babies would get to meet their mommies. (If you are not shedding a tear right now, I'll try harder, later.)

It is not just the major deficiencies in thyroid hormone during the second trimester that worry me, it is the subtle deficiency of thyroid hormone, one that goes unnoticed and perturbs the developing brain, which is of great concern. Perhaps in an effort to do all it can to prevent thyroid hormone deficiency or to limit its severity, the fetus has a clever little trick up its sleeve.

By the end of the first trimester, the fetus begins to swallow the surrounding amniotic fluid, actually snacking on it in order to obtain nutrients and other substances necessary for growth and development (Wikipedia, 2014). (If my memory serves me well, it didn't taste too bad.) What may come as a complete surprise is that the amniotic fluid is chock full of thyroid hormone! (Huang et al., 2003) This is its secret stash! Although when times are tough, *this* may not be enough. Nevertheless, the fetus swallows about two cups of amniotic fluid a day. Presumably, this beverage may become low in thyroid hormone and may fail to deliver on its promise to help satisfy the thyroid hormone needs of the developing fetus.

That's enough for the time being. You get the point. As in the first trimester of pregnancy, thyroid hormone should be in adequate supply during this second trimester or problems, sometimes big problems, could arise. Now on to the home stretch! And I do mean "stretch"—just wait and see how big a tummy can get! We'll find out how big in the next trimester.

The third trimester

> *From the second trimester onward, the major adverse obstetrical outcome associated with raised TSH in general population is an increased rate of fetal death.*   ~**Allan et al., 2000**

Only three long, challenging months to go! "When will that nursery <u>ever</u> be finished?" "Will I be able to fit through the door?" **"Will I explode?"** Frequently, these questions are raised. Neurons are being formed at the rate of **25,000 per minute!** The formation of the inner ear will take place (thyroid problems that occur during this time may cause irreversible hearing loss (Wasserman et al., 2007). Mom is worried when the fetus takes a break from kicking her all the time. The eyes are now fully formed. And the fetus is now practicing blinking, presumably in preparation for the time when cameras will be a-flashin'. This baby is kinda ready for the world, but a premature birth is not a good idea, no, not at all! In fact, it's a lousy idea. Should this occur, problems with the sudden loss of the mother's thyroid hormone contribution can develop and put the early arrival at serious risk. This spells trouble. And any degree of hypothyroxinemia previously experienced by the individual under construction is certain to be compounded.

Aside from the threat of prematurity, the fetus faces a number of challenges related to thyroid hormone availability. For example, the fetus will need to accumulate iodine in its little thyroid gland so that it can sustain thyroid hormone production after birth. The newborn only has a limited amount of iodine on board, even under the best of circumstances, and will soon run low if postnatal iodine intake is insufficient. Then, he or she will be at risk of developing hypothyroidism from iodine deficiency, and at a time his or her brain is still under construction (Akinci et al., 2006; Ghirri et al., 2014). Bad things happen to little babies when they are not up to the task of providing themselves with adequate amounts of thyroid hormone shortly after birth (Akinci et al., 2006). Iodine, received via breast milk from an adequately supplemented mother or via formula is, therefore, most essential (Ghirri et al., 2014). The new baby will need an adequate iodine intake in order to make enough thyroid hormone to continue the task of further development. This is why Mom's iodine intake should be even higher when breastfeeding than the amount recommended during pregnancy (Dunn and Delange, 2001). But look at me! I've jumped the gun. That cute little baby of yours, the one with an amazing brain (I'm crossing my fingers), has not yet been born!

The fourth trimester

Well, <u>this</u> trimester will end soon, very soon (let's hope)— things have gone on ... **way** ... **too** ... **long!** Inducing the delivery, or undergoing C-section, are strong possibilities. Mom is very big and wants to become smaller, rapidly (before she actually does explode)—and will soon be very glad when this ordeal is all over.

(Small, traumatic, and somewhat messy time lapse)

Now the moment all have been eagerly waiting for has arrived. The baby is finally here (and kinda ugly for the moment)! Cigars that should <u>never</u> be lit are being passed out! And, dad? Boy did he have a rough go of it! Not to worry! He will eventually recover from the trauma of birth.

The best of the best

Pregnancy is truly an amazing event. To see how amazing, you should read the following two books:

—*A Child is Born*, by Lennart Nilssan

—*The Miraculous World of Your Unborn Baby*, by Kikki Bradford

Chapter 3
What *ever* could go wrong?

In the USA 60% of pregnancies are unplanned, 16% of women do not receive prenatal care until the second trimester and 4% do not have prenatal care. **~Glinoer and Smallridge, 2004**

Pregnancy is a period that places great physiological stress on both the mother and the fetus. When pregnancy is complicated by endocrine disorders such as hypothyroidism, the potential for maternal and fetal adverse outcomes can be immense. **~Sahay and Sir Negesh, 2012**

*A growing body of clinical and experimental evidence indicates that **even slight decreases** in serum [blood] levels of THs [thyroid hormones] can have significant consequences on brain development.* **~Nucera, 2010, emphasis added**

Maternal thyroid insufficiency in early pregnancy, including clinical hypothyroidism, subclinical hypothyroidism, and hypothyroxinemia, may lead to delayed brain development and intellectual retardation in the fetus. It may also increase the incidence of complications such as miscarriage, premature labor, preeclampsia, breech delivery, and fetal death. **~Yu et al., 2013**

Let me tell you what can go wrong. A lot can go wrong. During pregnancy, even if the thyroid status of the mother is off just a little, trouble can ensue (Nucera, 2010). *"Even slight decreases"* in thyroid hormone availability can negatively affect the developing brain (Yu et al., 2013). And don't think thyroid abnormalities are rare during pregnancy. *"Thyroid diseases affect up to 5% of all pregnancies."* (Männistö, 2013, emphasis added) To put this another way, **up to 1 out of every 20** women you know who are currently pregnant or who have recently been pregnant, has or has had a thyroid-related problem during pregnancy. **It's not rare!** No, not at all. It is way too common and places in jeopardy the outcome of many a pregnancy. (Kids arrive damaged, if they arrive at all.)

Next, let's take a look at what can go wrong when the maternal iodine, and most particularly, when the maternal thyroid status is *"off just a little"* (or off just a lot). We're talkin' trouble!

Iodine deficiency

The mother and fetus must have adequate iodine throughout the pregnancy. Screening for maternal hypothyroidism during pregnancy should be strongly considered, particularly in areas of iodine deficiency, even if borderline. **~Dunn and Delange, 2001**

The fetus is particularly vulnerable to damage from iodine deficiency early in pregnancy, and if supplementation begins only at the first prenatal care visit, this critical period may be missed. **~Zimmermann and Delange, 2004**

*A **50% increase in iodine intake is recommend** in order for pregnant women to produce enough thyroid hormones to meet fetal requirements. A lack of iodine in the diet may result in the mother becoming deficient, and subsequently the fetus.* **~Skeaff, 2011, emphasis added**

Furthermore and importantly, among the women aged 15–45 yrs, 5–12% had a UIC [urinary iodine concentration] below 50

µg/L. . . . Thus, the iodine nutrition status is probably marginally restricted or even moderately deficient in a non-negligible fraction of the "to-be-pregnant" female population in the United States.
~Glinoer and Smallridge, 2004

We will be brief in this section, as this subject will be covered in greater depth later in the following two chapters. But let's take a quick look at iodine and the negative effects of its deficiency during pregnancy.

Iodine is such a little thing. A tiny little atom, but *essential* to normal embryonic/fetal development. How essential, you ask?

Iodine deficiency rarely produces malformations identifiable at birth, but it interferes severely with prenatal and postnatal growth and neurological development of individuals. It condemns millions of children to cretinism, tens of millions to mental retardation, and hundreds of millions to milder degrees of mental and physical impairments. (Hollowell and Hannon, 1997)

Iodine deficiency increases neonatal mortality. We emphasize this statement so that iodine deficiency can take its proper place among the disorders that kill children. (Dunn and Delange, 2001)

Very important must it be, this iodine atom—actually, life-and-death important! It is extremely important for the quality of life a child will have later on. Mom, you're going to need a lot of these things around to pull off a successful pregnancy and to get your baby off to a good start. As promised, we will talk more about iodine later, much more, but I need to add this to the present discussion before I forget:

In America—a region generally considered to be iodine sufficient—the prevalence of iodine deficiency is about **1 in 10** individuals (Klubo-Gwiezdzinska et al., 2011). Unfortunately, there is no real test that reflects the iodine stores and the day-by-day sufficiency of an individual's iodine status. There are just too many variables. And thyroid hormone levels may not offer any clue, as they may be normal even when an individual is, indeed, iodine deficient (Morreale de Escobar et al., 2007).

In the case of <u>mild to moderate</u> iodine deficiency during the pregnancy, the circulating T3 levels remain normal or even increase slightly and circulating TSH levels do not increase. So the thyroid function tests may misleadingly indicate euthyroidism, while the amount of T4 available for the fetus might be insufficient. (Klubo-Gwiezdzinska et al., 2011, emphasis added)

So much of this madness could be prevented if only we did not assume that we, as a nation, were iodine sufficient, and, accordingly, we did something to correct the problem of iodine deficiency and take it completely out of the picture. We especially need to direct our focus on women in their childbearing years, the pregnant and potentially pregnant ladies in our midst. This is sure to have its rewards.

Iodine supplementation from conception will ensure adequate FT4 during all of gestation and lactation; especially up to midgestation when the fetal brain is particularly vulnerable to iodine deficiency. (Berbel et al., 2009)

Reliance on the TSH

*In pregnant women thyroid and pituitary functions are not stable, and, therefore, measuring TSH is not sufficient and often inappropriate for the assessment of thyroid hormone during gestation. **If serum TSH measurement is used alone, the mother*** *is likely to be insufficiently treated . . . .   ~Feldt-Rasmussen et al., 2011, emphasis added*

I don't want to tarnish the reputation of the TSH test (actually I do, but not tarnish it too much), it certainly has its place in guiding therapy and in screening for abnormalities, but it is <u>not</u> the final word on . . . **anything!** To assume otherwise is a precarious position to take. What the research clearly shows is that, during pregnancy, a reliance <u>only</u> on the TSH (to determine if all is well from a thyroid hormone standpoint) can often be misleading, giving the impression that there is certain to be enough T4 around when this may not be the case. Some little someone could get hurt (damaged) by not receiving his or her fair share. And the crazy thing is this damage can occur while the TSH is saying that "all is well." (If you forgot what the TSH is, please see the gray box at the end of the *Introduction*) But more than the TSH is needed for more informative screening.

What is also needed is some kind of T4 estimate, either a free T4 (*f*T4), a total T4 level, or a T4-estimate calculation of some sort—<u>anything</u> that will give the physician a clue as to the ability of the mother to deliver on the promise of supplying enough T4 to meet the developmental needs of her baby (Feldt-Rasmussen et al., 2011). As a patient, you can request a more complete thyroid workup, other than a basic TSH lab draw. Requesting (insisting on) a *f*T4 level (and a TSH) is a good call. Why? Along with a TSH, a *f*T4 level in hand is the standard test used to identify the following <u>serious</u> medical condition.

Hypothyroxinemia

*Hypothyroxinemia [remember, "low T4"] is a **common condition** in pregnant women. It is characterized by low maternal*

*free thyroid hormone (fT4) concentrations with thyrotropin (TSH)
concentrations in the normal range. This condition has long been
regarded as being without consequences for mother and fetus
[**Oops!**].* ~Kooistra et al., 2006, emphasis added

*Maternal hypothyroxinemia is an asymptomatic condition
for the mother, but it is <u>extremely</u> harmful for the fetus. Because
the fetus's thyroid is still too immature to synthesize sufficient T3
and T4, the fetus relies on the maternal thyroid hormone for its
optimal brain development.* ~Opazo et al., 2008, emphasis
added

*A 50% increase in iodine intake is recommend in order for
pregnant women to produce enough thyroid hormones to meet
fetal requirements. A lack of iodine in the diet may result in the
mother becoming deficient, and subsequently the fetus. **The
mother and the fetus, however, respond differently to this
situation, with the mother remaining euthroid [considered as
having normal thyroid function] and the fetus becoming
hypothyroid.*** ~Skeaff, 2011, emphasis added

*Most cases of maternal hypothyroxinemia are related to a
relative iodine deficiency during pregnancy that can be so easily
prevented, with minimal expense, without risk and with worldwide
success.* ~Morreale de Escobar et al., 2004, emphasis added

What is hypothyroxinemia and why is it bad? I have shared
this with your before. Hypothyroxinemia is a deficiency of T4 in
the bloodstream. It is bad is because it limits the amount of T4
that can be delivered to the one who is developing inside.
Remember this well: <u>**Hypothyroxinemia in the mother creates
hypothyroidism in the baby.**</u> What I may not have shared with
you previously is that *hypothyroxinemia occurs when the TSH is
normal!* The reason why the TSH is normal is because, in this
condition, thyroidal T3 production becomes elevated and makes
the pituitary gland think and act as if all is well (when it is not),

hence the TSH will not be elevated even though the T4 level is low. Let's look a little deeper.

A normal TSH generally means that the pituitary thinks the individual's thyroid hormone status is satisfactory, and does not feel it necessary to increase its production of TSH in order to "force" the thyroid gland to respond and increase production of more thyroid hormone, both T3 and T4.

In the case of hypothyroxinemia, a deception is taking place. The TSH suggests nothing is wrong, but T4 is actually in short supply. Recall, the embryo/fetus needs little if any T3 from Mom, it wants T4. Maternal hypothyroxinemia, therefore, stands directly in the way. It is a chronic deficiency in T4, a situation creating a failure to supply enough T4 to meet the needs of the one who is developing inside. This is why it is bad. This is why hypothyroxinemia can damage the brain. This is why it can *really* damage the brain, such as is seen in cerebral palsy. That's how bad it is. Very bad. And did I mention that hypothyroxinemia is deceptive? And did I mention that hypothyroxinemia is not rare? *"While the incidence of hypothyroidism in pregnant women is around 2.5%, hypothyroxinemia is much more prevalent, **up to 30%**, and it is usually due to mild iodine deficiency."* (Bernal, 2014, emphasis added) Notice the words *"mild iodine deficiency"*—very important. Mildly iodine-deficient ladies are everywhere!

So here's the problem: If only a TSH level is checked at the first prenatal visit, hypothyroxinemia, if it does indeed exist, will be missed. The TSH will not inform of this serious medical condition. It takes another test to identify hypothyroxinemia. The test is called a free T4 (*f*T4), and its use (or the use of a similar test) is necessary to diagnose this abnormality. If this second test is not performed, the deception continues and jeopardizes everything. And an adverse pregnancy outcome, when it does occur, may not be attributed to maternal hypothyroxinemia . . . ever, as no one became, or will become, aware of its existence in that mother in question . . . ever! That's how deceptive it is, and it has the power to damage lives today just as it has so many times in the past. Millions of lives have been seriously harmed or destroyed by hypothyroxinemia.

Hypothyroxinemia is typically caused by iodine deficiency, a deficiency which commonly occurs throughout the world, even in iodine sufficient countries (Morreale de Escobar et al., 2004; Verheesen and Schweitzer, 2008). All a mother needs to be is "mildly iodine deficient" for problems to occur (Bernal, 2014).

Here's what happens in hypothyroxinemia: When the thyroid gland does not obtain enough iodine, it enlarges. Over time, a goiter develops—an ominous sign that a serious problem exists, and has for quite some time. The thyroid gland is increasing in size in order to extract more iodine from the bloodstream. Typically, a goiter is a signal that iodine intake has been insufficient . . . long term (Ghirri et al., 2014). And a chronic lack of iodine in Mom can cause devastating effects to her unborn baby. **Remember this well: Due to a deficiency in iodine, the mother's thyroid will produce an excess of T3 at the expense of producing an adequate amount of T4.** *"Under circumstances of sustained iodine deficiency, a shift in T3/T4 balance will occur in favor of T3."* (Verheesen and Schweitzer, 2008) Due to iodine deficiency in Mom some little someone is at great risk of improper development due to a lack of T4, due to hypothyroxinemia. All I can say at this point is *"Yikes!"* Now with that little outburst out of the way, we can continue.

"And tell me again, why do we want to detect hypothyroxinemia?" you ask. I can share *this* with you:

Nelson and Ellenberg report that children of women who were **hypothyroxinemic or hyperthyroxinemic** <u>both before or during pregnancy</u> may have poor fine motor coordination, varying degrees of mental retardation, specific signs of cerebral palsy (including spasticity, tone abnormalities, and hemiparesis), and a **<u>20-fold increase</u> of risk for later cerebral palsy.** (Hollowell and Hannon, 1997, emphasis added)

Every effort must be made to detect and prevent early maternal hypothyroxinemia to prevent neurodevelopmental defects, which may include an increased chance of a lower IQ and a higher risk of **cerebral palsy.** (Negro et al., 2006, emphasis added)

There are a multitude of <u>great</u> reasons to detect and to correct hypothyroxinemia, ASAP. This is one *very* deceptive medical condition. And the deception extends to how a pregnant lady, or potentially pregnant lady, feels. She feels great! (Except for the fact that they may feel like crap for various other reasons.) Hypothyroxinemia is asymptomatic (and so willing to deceive). It is <u>not</u> hypothyroidism in Mom, per se—the extra T3 onboard prevents that. It is, however, hypothyroidism for the fetus. *"Every effort"* should be made to detect it! And you can only detect it by measuring a free T4 level (or similar test) in Mom and finding it to be low when the TSH is normal. May I repeat? **If the TSH is the only thyroid screening lab drawn, hypothyroxinemia will be missed, should it exist.** And a deception may turn into a tragedy.

I suppose, if a clinician is inclined not to treat it, there is no reason to look for it. So, currently, I see little effort put forth to detect or treat hypothyroxinemia. But, in as much as iodine deficiency is the leading cause of this disorder, detecting hypothyroxinemia would certainly invite close attention to the iodine status of the mother-to-be. Even in geographical areas where iodine deficiency is endemic (therefore hypothyroxinemia is endemic), *"iodine supplementation to women before pregnancy or up to the end of the second trimester protects the fetal brain from the effects of iodine deficiency."* (Ogilvy-Stuart, 2002) But the earlier, the better! It has been reported that a *"delay of 6–10 weeks in iodine supplementation of hypothyroxinemia mothers at the beginning of gestation increases the risk of neurodevelopmental delay in the progeny."* (Berbel et al., 2009)

Let me close out this section with this: If you do not know what cerebral palsy is, good for you! I wish I didn't know what it is. I take care of individuals with cerebral palsy from time to time in my nursing practice. I know why some of them develop this condition, it rips my heart out, and I can no longer remain on the sidelines. The belief that careful screening of the thyroid hormone status of each mother-to-be is unnecessary is one cause of cerebral palsy, and a preventable one at that. Approximately 764,000 Americans have cerebral palsy in varying degrees, with 8,000 to 10,000 added to the list yearly, so this is not that rare of a condition. (source: CerebralPalsy.Org) Actually, hypothyroxinemia is not a rare condition. It effects one in every—well, we just don't know. Because so many pregnant women are not tested, or tested only with a TSH (often normal regardless of the presence of a thyroid disease or imbalance), the true prevalence of this disorder is a big unknown. **Its incidence during pregnancy may be as high as 30% of all pregnancies** (Bernal, 2014).

Subclinical hypothyroidism

Our observations add to accruing data that subclinical hypo-thyroidism, a relatively common finding in women of childbearing age, may be associated with some adverse perinatal outcomes.

Women with subclinical hypothyroidism identified during pregnancy have an increased risk for severe preeclampsia when compared to euthyroid women. **~Wilson et al., 2012**

Subclinical hypothyroidism is defined as increased TSH with normal concentrations of FT4 and FT3. The prevalence of subclinical hypothyroidism is estimated to be 2% to 5%. It is almost always asymptomatic. **~Sahay and Nagesh, 2012**

Even mild or subclinical maternal hypothyroidism during pregnancy can impair mental development of the newborn. **~Zimmermann and Delange, 2004**

In comparison to euthyroid controls, women with sub-clinical hypothyroidism (an elevated TSH and normal T4 concentration) experienced a 3-fold increase in placental abruption and a 2-fold increase in preterm birth. **~Alexander, 2010**

This thyroid hormone condition, subclinical hypothyroidism, is also deceptive. Here you have an elevated TSH, but the T3 and T4 levels are within normal limits. This basically means that the thyroid gland is being flogged a little (chemically, by TSH stimulation) in order to perform. I feel sorry for the thyroid gland at times—so much is riding on it being able to fulfill its obligations. But in subclinical hypothyroidism the T4 level is supposedly "normal," so what's the big deal? There are a couple of good explanations why this condition is harmful in the context of pregnancy.

First, although "normal," the T4 level may be too low for the baby developing inside (Adlin, 1998,; Ausó et al., 2004). Indeed, in subclinical hypothyroidism *"the increased TSH indicates that thyroidal hormone production is already inadequate for that person, even if circulating concentration are within the very broadly normal range."* (Ausó et al., 2004) **Second**, an individual with subclinical hypothyroidism is much more likely to have antithyroid antibodies floating around in the bloodstream (Sahay and Negesh, 2012). Antithyroid antibodies can cause all sorts of havoc for the fetus and can even lead to pregnancy loss, which means baby loss (Thangaratinam et al., 2011).

> The one salient finding of this study that included nearly 25,000 pregnant women was that those identified to have subclinical hypothyroidism had a significantly increased risk for development of severe preeclampsia when compared with euthyroid women. (Wilson et al., 2012)

Babies are lost when severe preeclampsia strikes. Mothers can also be lost. Subclinical hypothyroidism is <u>not</u> benign, it is evil. *"Even subclinical hypothyroidism . . . has been shown to be associated with an adverse outcome for both the mother and her offspring."* (Matuszek et al., 2011) *"Allan et al., in 2000, demonstrated that pregnant women with TSH levels greater than 6.0 mIU/L had a significantly higher rate of fetal death than controls."* (Cignini et al., 2012) Furthermore, one group of investigators found that *"pregnancies in women with subclinical hypothyroidism were 3 times more likely to be complicated by placental abruption."* (Casey et al., 2005)

When it comes to the advisability of treating subclinical hypothyroidism, the jury is still out (which means, people are still dragging their feet).

> Treatment of subclinical hypothyroidism during pregnancy is not universally recommended however a recent paper by Negro et al. has shown that treatment

reduces the occurrence of adverse outcomes in the mother and fetus. (Ghirri et al., 2013)

Next, let's take a little break. This stuff is not at all what you are used to studying. But keep in mind, learning this may make all the difference in both your future and that of your baby. I didn't promise learning this would be easy—well, maybe I did. But you can get this! It just may take a couple readings of this chapter to understand what the heck is going on. **Hint:** What the heck is going on is that thyroid problems interfere with normal fetal development by limiting the availability of T4 to meet the needs of the one who is developing inside. What else is going on is that the pregnant mother's thyroid status is often, very often, not investigated thoroughly enough to identify all the thyroid-related threats facing both mother and baby. We need to change this. We can change this. Now, enjoy the break.

(Short, pleasant time lapse)

Now that you are back and refreshed from our little break, let's move on. I see more trouble ahead.

Hypothyroidism

*It is estimated that 3–7% of women of childrearing age are hypothyroid. Although some are undiagnosed, most hypothyroid women have been identified and are receiving T4. Because greater than 4 million live births occur annually in the United States, **some 100,000–200,000 women and their unborn fetuses are at risk** and require a reliable, clinically tested strategy to treat this condition. Presently, most women first receive obstetrical care during their 8–12 week of pregnancy. Although relatively* *early, this is late for hypothyroid women . . . .*   **~Yassa et al., 2010, emphasis added**

Many women with pre-existing hypothyroidism are diagnosed and treated with supplemental T4, but the majority of these women tend to be under-treated because their T4 doses are not increased to match the normal physiological demands for TH [thyroid hormone] during pregnancy.   **~Wilson et al., 2012**

One possible approach is to instruct hypothyroid women to increase their T4 dosage upon initial diagnosis of pregnancy. This would allow a window of safety until more formal medical evaluation can be provided.   **~Yassa et al., 2010**

Hypothyroidism is what we generally think of when we think of thyroid hormone deficiency.   Basically, in hypothyroidism the thyroid gland is crippled in its efforts to produce enough thyroid hormone for its owner, let alone for anyone else.   It takes approximately a **20–40%** increase in T4 production to meet the demands of pregnancy (Yassa et al., 2010). This is serious business. Pregnancy loss or a wide range of adverse fetal outcomes may result from maternal hypothyroidism (and its undertreatment). TSH levels above 6 mU/l, a level that would clearly indicate hypothyroidism, are *"significantly associated with a higher frequency of stillbirth."* (Benhadi et al., 2009) *"Even in healthy women without overt thyroid dysfunction, there is an increased risk of miscarriage, fetal death or neonatal death with increasing levels of TSH in pregnancy."* (Benhadi et al., 2009)

I am not alone in holding the following belief: It is imperative to screen every pregnant woman as soon as possible for thyroid hormone abnormalities (best before the pregnancy begins). Any abnormality discovered, even minor, should place the woman on her physician's radar screen, and frequent follow-up testing is more likely to be performed. And here's a twist: The presence of antithyroid antibodies (more next section) can lead to overt thyroid failure as a pregnancy progresses, particularly by what are called TPO antibodies (Feldt-Rasmussen et al., 2011). This is trouble! Be on the lookout! Early detection and prompt treatment followed by monthly thyroid testing may be in order (Männistö, 2013). By not testing timely and appropriately, or by not testing at all, opportunities are missed to prevent complications and unfavorable outcomes—and their occurrence is generally never traced back to thyroid hormone issues that went completely unnoticed during the pregnancy.

Insufficient thyroid hormone replacement

Women with hypothyroidism treated insufficiently with levothyroxine . . . deliver babies with significantly lower IQ and/or other inhibited neuropsychological development. Such offspring outcomes has even been demonstrated in women with a serum concentration of T4 in the low normal range during pregnancy.
~Feldt-Rasmussen et al., 2011

When hypothyroidism exists in the mother-to-be, the right dosage of thyroid replacement will need to be prescribed. Even before pregnancy occurs, in a planned pregnancy the best approach appears to be increasing the dosage of T4, perhaps by a tablet or two extra per week (Yassa et al., 2010). Pregnancy, once in progress, will automatically increase the demand for T4, yet without an associated increase in the maintenance dosage of T4 the embryo/fetus may simply not get enough T4 to meet its needs. This was not always understood.

Once upon a time, in the not-too-distant past, it was believed that the mother should stop her thyroid hormone therapy during pregnancy. Well, all I can say is **"Yikes!"**

This is a very important issue that has, unfortunately, been somewhat misunderstood for decades, to the point that Mesterman unexpectedly found that in a recent study [1999] from Los Angeles involving 78 women who were hypothyroid at booking into the clinic, 34 (44%) had discontinued therapy [T4 hormonal replacement] at the time they discovered they were pregnant "some after receiving advice from their own health care professionals, and others because of concern for the potential harmful effect of thyroid medications on the conceptus [developing embryo/fetus and supporting structures]." (Morreale de Escobar et al., 2000, emphasis added)

We know better now! For those with hypothyroidism, the thyroid hormone dose should be increased during pregnancy, not decreased, not stopped, and not ignored. The undertreatment of hypothyroidism in hypothyroid mommies is, to the fetus, the gift of hypothyroidism. I can only imagine the harm that occurred to past generations of babies when Mom followed the unfortunate advice to stop thyroid hormone therapy during pregnancy. Say it with me, *"Yikes!"*

Perhaps surprisingly, there is another way to be undertreated: Right medicine, right dose, but Mom is taking her thyroid medication at the same time she is taking her newly prescribed iron/calcium-rich prenatal vitamin tablet. **OMG!** Was Mom not warned that the iron and calcium in her prenatal will bind with her thyroid medication and interfere with its absorption? (Ozdemir et al., 2013) This mistake—taking a prenatal vitamin with thyroid hormone medication—may reduce the availability of T4 to meet the needs of the one who is counting on Mom not to screw up here. If frequent testing is not performed, a low T4 level may go unnoticed for quite some time or may never come to the attention of the physician and corrective action may never be taken.

Autoimmune thyroid disease

In developed countries, the most common cause of thyroid disorder in women of reproductive age is autoimmune thyroid disease.

Ten to 20% of pregnant women have anti-thyroid antibodies as do 1/10 of newborn infants. ~Nelson, 2009, emphasis added

Elevated maternal thyroid autoantibodies during pregnancy are linked to infertility, miscarriage, and neurodevelopmental defects such as in cognitive function. ~**Wasserman et al., 2007**

Autoimmune thyroid disorders have been associated with an increased risk for placental abruption [separation]. ~**Wilson et al., 2012**

Indeed, in our series [a study of 220 women living in a mild iodine deficient region] . . . thyroid autoimmunity carried a 5-fold increased risk of hypothyroidism. ~**Moleti et al., 2009**

*Stagnaro-Green et al. reported a statistically significant **doubling in the miscarriage rate** in American euthyroid women in the first trimester of pregnancy who were thyroid antibody positive.* ~**Stagnaro-Green, 2011, emphasis added**

Perhaps the best way to describe thyroid autoimmune disease is to compare it to what we do when we deal with bacteria that have invaded. Our immune cells attack 'em and destroy 'em. In the case of autoimmune thyroid disease, there is an antibody attack on normal thyroid cells or related proteins.

An antibody is a molecule that attaches to a foreign cell such as a bacterium, interferes with its function, and marks it for destruction—annihilation by an immune cell designed for this task. Antibodies also mistakenly attack our own cells under certain circumstances. They can interfere with, attack, and destroy thyroid cells and certain proteins involved in the thyroid hormone economy. This occurs slowly, and over time hypothyroidism developes. Watch out!

Autoimmune thyroid disease can be found in **1 out of 8** pregnancies in North America (Ozdemir et al., 2013). *1 out of 8! OMG!* Indeed, *"Thyroid autoantibodies are detected in about 50% of pregnant women with subclinical hypothyroidism, and in 80% of those women with clinical hypothyroidism."* (Obican et al., 2012, emphasis added) And as a result, *"thyroid function deteriorates into subclinical hypothyroidism in women with thyroid autoimmunity."* (Seror et al., 2014) Or the following may occur: *"pregnant women with positive antibodies are more prone to develop hypothyroxinemia."* (Hendrichs et al., 2010)

I sure hope thyroid autoimmunity is not present in your pregnancy, undetected, unaddressed, and problematic. Thyroid autoimmunity, leading to subclinical hypothyroidism later in the pregnancy, may produce a *f*T4 level *"30% lower compared with those women who are antibody-negative."* (Seror et al., 2014, emphasis added) I see a big problem here! The thyroid antibody status of the mother-to-be needs to be investigated, positive vs. negative, and without delay. Indeed,

> Because euthyroid women with features of thyroid autoimmunity are at risk of developing hypothyroidism during pregnancy, they should be monitored for an increase in serum TSH. Subclinical hypothyroidism is associated with

an adverse outcome in pregnancy. (Glinoer and Abalovich, 2007)

Many, perhaps most, clinics in the USA only test the TSH at the first prenatal visit, and if the TSH is normal, further investigation of a mother's thyroid status will not be forthcoming. Unfortunately, a TSH will not and cannot detect the presence of thyroid autoimmunity. This problem will be missed and will <u>never</u> be identified as the cause of an unfortunate outcome related to unidentified autoimmunity against the thyroid. "Someone" is not practicing preventative medicine, at least not as well as those who are faithfully checking their patients for antithyroid antibodies before conception or as soon as possible during the pregnancy. Am I being too harsh? The answer to follow.

No. I'm not being too harsh. One reason antithyroid antibodies should be checked as soon as possible during pregnancy is because the mother with this disorder has a **60 to 70% risk of becoming hypothyroid later in her pregnancy** (Feldt-Rasmussen et al., 2011). This late-onset hypothyroidism, too, may be missed—*missed!*—if we assume a normal TSH at the beginning of pregnancy will remain normal throughout the entire pregnancy. Not only is the existence of antithyroid antibodies a problem in and of itself, but the partial destruction of the mother's thyroid gland can mean low levels of thyroid hormone available to share with little Jimmy or little Susie, or whomever the little guy or gal will eventually turn into (Wasserman et al., 2007). I don't even what to think of another pregnancy that may occur soon after the pregnancy that is currently underway. The subsequent pregnancy, too, may be adversely affected should this late-onset hypothyroidism not be identified and corrected during the pregnancy currently underway.

So, what can be done in the context of thyroid autoimmunity? The physician can protect the pregnancy, protect the baby—protect the future—by prescribing T4, as indicated, and following the mother's thyroid status very closely. Consider this:

> The rate of spontaneous miscarriage was 13.8% in untreated thyroid antibody positive women and 2.4% in the 890 controls. Thyroid antibody positive women who received levothyroxine [T4] had a spontaneous miscarriage rate of 3.5% which was similar to controls [those without thyroid antibodies] (2.4%), and statistically lower than the miscarriage rate in the untreated thyroid antibody positive controls [those positive who received no treatment]. (Stagnaro-Green, 2011)

One reason—the best reason—to screen for antithyroid antibodies is to save babies from death before birth. Clearly, treatment with T4 can save babies when the mother's immune system has gone over to the dark side. The TSH, in this situation, can serve as a guide. If over 2.5, T4 replacement therapy may be advised (Stagnaro-Green, 2011).

> Negro et al., in a pioneering study, found that LT4 administration in euthyroid women with autoimmune thyroid disease decreased the rates of negative obstetric outcomes in women with a TSH value greater than 2.0 mLU/liter and/or a high titer of thyroid antibodies. (Sahay and Nagesh, 2012)

One negative obstetric outcome, surprisingly related to thyroid autoimmunity, is hearing loss. Hearing loss in the baby can occur due to the maternal transfer of antithyroid antibodies present during a critical time during fetal development when inner ear formation takes center stage (Wasserman et al, 2007). Are you listening? Thyroid autoimmunity leads to some very unfortunate things. Several unfortunate things readily come to mind.

For example, *"pregnant women with positive antibodies are more prone to developing hypo-thyroxinemia."* (Hendrichs et al., 2010) As we have previously discussed, hypothyroxinemia—a deficiency in T4 when the TSH says all is well—damages babies. In fact, *"it is extremely harmful for the fetus."* (Opazo et al., 2008)

Given all we know of the dangers—given all that is at stake!—we should be screening for and treating autoimmune thyroid disease in ladies who make babies.

> TPOaAB positivity may not only predict an increased risk of clinical thyroid disease in the women themselves but also mark <u>preventable</u> neurodevelopmental defects in their children. (Wasserman et al., 2007, emphasis added)

We really need to look. We really need to know.

> **During pregnancy autoimmunity damage to the maternal thyroid gland may <u>critically</u> reduce the supply of maternal thyroid hormones to the offspring.** (Hendrichs et al., 2013, emphasis added)

Do not fool around with not looking. Don't fool around with not knowing. Find out for sure. Insist! I am not the only one who wants you to be tested to see if you are antithyroid antibody positive.

Prematurity

Infants born prematurely tend to have hypothyroxinemia and are also at risk of neurologic and developmental problems.
~Reuss et al., 1996

Hypothyroxinemia affects 35–50% of neonates born prematurely (12% of births) and increases their risk of suffering neurodevelopmental alterations.   **~Berbel et al., 2010**

*Scientists have linked low levels of a thyroid hormone in premature infants to the development of disabling cerebral palsy. They examined more than 400 premature infants screened for blood levels of the hormone thyroxin during the first week of life. They found that <u>infants with low levels of thyroxin at birth had a</u> <u>**3- to 4-fold increase**</u> <u>in the incidence of</u> **cerebral palsy** <u>at age 2.</u>*
~National Institute of Neurological Disorders and Stroke, 1996, emphasis added

On several levels, prematurity is bad news. It represents a level of immaturity that may challenge the health and survival of the new little arrival, and challenge for days, weeks, months, and years . . . even for a lifetime! Immediately, a premature birth severs the connection between mother and baby. No more thyroid hormone from Mom for little Jimmy or little Susie! No more amniotic fluid to swallow! Ready or not, the new baby will have to rely upon his or her own production of thyroid hormone. I sure hope the little one is up to the task. (But he or she won't be if he or she is iodine deficient.) But the unfortunate fact is that because of iodine deficiency many do not have the ability to do meet their need for thyroid hormone and, therefore, will continue their development under the cloud of hypothyroxinemia or hypothyroidism.

On the surface, it appears that little can be done from a thyroid hormone standpoint, as prematurity creates a unique set of circumstances that may actually make thyroid hormone supplementation harmful (Ogilvy-Stuart, 2002). Controversy still exists whether preterm babies should be treated with thyroid hormone (Bernal, 2014). So we usually ride out the storm and hope for the best.

Prematurity is simply a bad idea. Every effort should be made to prevent it. *"In this country, preterm birth is overwhelmingly the most common recognized cause of neuropsychologic dysfunction in children."* (Casey et al., 2005) Prematurity places your baby at increased risk of developmental delay, of autism, of cerebral palsy, of schizophrenia, of so many things you want to avoid at all costs. One problem is, if the iodine and thyroid hormone status of the mother is compromised—**and this goes unidentified**—the baby is already deficient in both iodine and T4 and may already be developmentally compromised. Furthermore, the premature baby may not have accumulated enough iodine in his or her little thyroid gland to rise to the challenge of manufacturing his or her own thyroid hormone in satisfactory amounts. In which case, a lack of iodine in Baby leads to hypothyroidism in Baby.

And with respect to iodine availability, *"Iodine deficiency is not only present in developing countries, but also widely spread in European countries and the USA."* (Verheesen and Schweitzer, 2008, emphasis added) Can you see why we have so many unfavorable pregnancy outcomes, clearly related to the iodine and thyroid hormone status of the mother during gestation, even apart from prematurity? Add prematurity to the mix, and the risk for an ensuing tragedy is amplified.

I'm going to add one more thing before we move on, trembling as we go. In a sense, even a timely birth can be a premature birth if the conditions are just right. If the new baby appears normal, with a normal screening TSH, he or she may fail to maintain adequate thyroid hormone production. The little thyroid gland is just not ready to perform. It may not have accumulated enough iodine, or it may be hampered by lingering antithyroid antibodies received from Mom during pregnancy, or both, and the new little one may become relatively hypothyroid in short order (Rastogi and LaFranchi, 2010). Sometimes a healthy little baby develops into a compromised little baby . . . and we wonder why.

I will throw this in now, even though I planned to share this with you later. If, for some reason, the new little arrival should be placed on a soy-based formula, I see trouble ahead and so does Dr. Román. Soy products, including soy-based formulas, contain components that interfere with thyroid hormone production and the uptake of iodine, potentially producing hypothyroidism in the new little baby (Román, 2007). Accordingly, its use in infant formula may make an already compromised thyroid hormone status compromised further. Thyroid hormone production may be impaired and may not be sufficient to sustain normal neurological development. A great deal of brain development occurs during the newborn period and during infancy (Akinci et al., 2006). Hypothyroidism in this period of life is not a good idea. Actually, it's a lousy idea. It can harm the brain. Up to 25% of infant formulas are soy-based, so there are many hungry little ones being placed at risk by something that appears so wholesome. If a soy-based formula is used, it should contain a satisfactory amount of iodine in order to reduce the tendency of soy to create goiter or hypothyroidism in the little one (Zimmermann, 2009). Food for thought.

Congenital hypothyroidism

Despite the success of neonatal screening programmes to identify and treat congenital hypothyroidism, in the newborn, these children still exhibit impairments. Their IQ levels average approximately 6 points below expectation and they also show selective deficits on visuospatial, motor, language, memory and attention tests. ~**Zoeller and Rovet, 2004**

Congenital hypothyroidism occurs when the baby's thyroid gland fails to develop normally, fails to function properly, or is absent entirely. Congenital hypothyroidism is, of course, a serious situation, now that the lifeline (umbilical cord) has been severed and the newborn has something new to swallow. This something new is called breast milk—tastes great! (I have an excellent memory.) Unfortunately, breast milk is low in thyroid hormone, and will not come to the aid of the new little one in this respect. And most unfortunately, in congenital hypothyroidism, Baby will have little or no thyroid hormone available to work with in short order, and at a time when having an adequate amount of thyroid hormone on board thyroid is underline critical to promote normal neurological development. This, of course, is very bad news. You don't need very bad news. But each and every year a thousand or more new mommies and daddies will hear the words "congenital hypothyroidism" for the first time. Let's see what this condition is all about.

As mentioned, congenital hypothyroidism can occur when the baby has no thyroid gland at all (Rastogi and LaFranchi, 2010). Or, sometimes it is due to a thyroid gland that is developmentally immature (Rastogi and LaFranchi, 2010). Alternatively, it can develop as a result of antithyroid antibodies—received from Mom—that are hanging around and interfering with neonatal thyroid hormone production (Rastogi and LaFranchi, 2010; Ghirri et al., 2013). Furthermore, congenital hypothyroidism can occur when Mom is taking too much iodine (Rastogi and LaFranchi, 2010). And sometimes it is caused by medications used to control Mom's hyperthyroidism (Rastogi and LaFranchi, 2010; Ghirri et al., 2013). But I have some good news to share (for a change).

Thankfully, every newborn is screened shortly after birth in order to identify this very condition, affecting 1 in every 2,000 to 4,000 live births (Rastogi and LaFranchi, 2010). Unfortunately, things can change after the initial evaluation has ruled out this disorder, and congenital hypothyroidism can rear its ugly head and go unnoticed (Rastogi and LaFranchi, 2010)— this is not common, but it sometimes happens. Perhaps it would be wise to re-screen newborn babies between two and six weeks of age to make sure that congenital hypothyroidism continues not to exist. (see Rastogi and LaFranchi, 2010) And the good news is: Congenital hypothyroidism is so easy to treat.

> Levothyroxin [T4] is the treatment of choice; the recommended starting dose is 10 to 15 mcg/kg/day. . . . Frequent laboratory monitoring in infancy is essential to ensure optimal neurocognitive outcome. Serum TSH should be measured every 1–2 months in the first 6 months of life and every 3–4 months thereafter. . . . Studies show that a lower neurocognitive outcome may occur in those infants started at a later age (> 30 days of age), on lower l-thyroxine [T4] doses that currently recommended, and in those infants with more severe hypothyroidism. (Rastogi and LaFranchi, 2010)

So, what should you look for that might suggest the existence of congenital hypothyroidism? If your newborn baby seems to be failing to thrive, there is at least some possibility that congenital hypothyroidism was missed or has somehow emerged. In any event, something is wrong—perhaps related to a thyroid hormone-related issue—and a reevaluation of baby's thyroid status is certainly in order.

> The clinical manifestations [of congenital hypo-thyroidism] are often subtle or not present at birth. This is likely due to trans-placental passage of some maternal thyroid hormone, while many infants have some thyroid production of their own. Common symptoms include decreased activity and increased sleep, feeding difficulty, constipation, and prolonged jaundice. (Rastogi and LaFranchi, 2010)

Let's move on. I see another problem I need to bring to your attention, without delay.

Hyperthyroidism

> *In recent analyses from a large US cohort, diagnosed hyperthyroidism (without data on treatment) increased risk of preeclampsia, preterm birth, labor inductions, maternal and neonatal intensive care unit admissions, neonatal respiratory diseases, sepsis, cardiomyopathy, retinopathy of prematurity and neonatal thyroid diseases.*

> *Hyperthyroidism is often treated with antithyroid drugs in pregnancy. However, they are not completely safe to use during pregnancy as methimazole increases risk of neonatal malformations . . . .* **~Männistö, 2013**

This will be a short section, as the focus of this book is on a lack of T4 during gestation and during postnatal life and not on the effects of thyroid hormone excess during pregnancy. But I need to point out a few things to keep in mind should you have hyperthyroidism. (Have you been screened to find out?)

In hyperthyroidism, the thyroid gland is producing too much thyroid hormone, both T3 and T4, and during pregnancy the fetus will have to deal with this excess. The placenta will respond and try her best (placentas are always girls) to filter out this excess, but "she" will not be able to prevent the fetus from excess exposure to T3 and T4. This challenges the developmental process and can be very harmful to the fetus. Birth defects can occur when Mom suffers from this disorder (Hollowell and Hannon, 1997). It can also be a cause of infertility or reproductive failure (Männistö, 2013; Hollowell and Hannon, 1997). Even if diagnosed and treated, the threat does not end.

Unfortunately, medical treatment of hyperthyroidism is not without risk and may lead to serious birth defects (Stagnaro-Green and Pearce, 2012; Männistö, 2013). Apparently, as in hypothyroxinemia, the fetus is not well served when Mom is sending way too much T3 its way. For normal development to occur little, if any, T3 is needed from Mom. And, the fetus only needs adequate amounts of T4 from Mom. Too much of either T3 or T4, or both, can spell trouble. By the way, the TSH excels in detecting hyperthyroidism. The TSH will be very low when hyperthyroidism exists.

This is one medical condition where it's probably time to call in a specialist. Its treatment during pregnancy should be expertly and carefully managed. And it does require treatment.

Hyperthyroidism is associated with increased risk of pregnancy complications, including miscarriages, preeclampsia, low birth weight or fetal growth restriction and maternal cardiac dysfunction, with risks increasing with poorer hyperthyroidism control. (Männistö, 2013)

One reason that careful management is a must when hyperthyroidism occurs during pregnancy is the medications used to control the disease can make the mother (hence, the fetus) hypothyroid. In one report, *"32% of women treated with ATDs [antithyroid drugs] alone became hypothyroid at some point during their pregnancy; in another report, the frequency of hypothyroidism defined by a low free T4 at term was 25%."* (Mandel and Cooper, 2001)

On a personal note: I have three lovely grand-nieces who would not be here today were it not for an observation made by my mother. One day, while visiting with her granddaughter, who was trying but could not get pregnant, my mother noticed that her granddaughter's eyes were a little "buggy." Knowing that this is a sign of hyperthyroidism, my mother suggested that she see her doctor right away and be tested for this disease. Sure enough, my niece did, indeed, have hyperthyroidism. Soon after treatment her lab values normalized and she became pregnant. Of course, one healthy baby was not enough. Two more healthy babies followed.

Word of advice: If you have or think you may have hyperthyroidism, get on this right away. Find an expert! Follow instructions to the letter. Some little someone may be counting on you.

Obesity

Research suggests that obesity during pregnancy slightly increases the risk of having a baby who's born with a birth defect, such as a problem with the heart or a condition affecting the brain or spinal cord (neural tube defect). ~**Mayo Clinic, 1998–2014**

Pregnancy is a time when *everything* should be examined just to see if any issues exist that may place the pregnancy and the developing fetus at risk. For many reasons, obesity plus pregnancy is a big red flag. A lot of problems here. A lot of everything here! *This* is a high risk pregnancy. But with great care the risks can be minimized. Apparently, obesity can alter thyroid hormone balance in favor of hypothyroxinemia. *"It has been observed that thyroid hormone levels are affected by BMI with higher TSH and FT3 and lower FT4 concentrations observed in obese women."* (Klubo-Gwiezdzinska et al., 2011) Hypothyroxinemia, as we have learned (please review), is *"extremely harmful"* to the developing fetus, and particularly harmful to the developing brain.

The bottom line in all of this: If you are significantly overweight, you have a greater risk of T4 insufficiency which, as we have discussed, will unfortunately add to the risks both you and your baby face. Careful monitoring of your thyroid status, and attention to iodine, both before and during pregnancy, is bordering on crucial. Let's just say it is crucial. Why place your baby at <u>any</u> unnecessary risk? And speaking of unnecessary risk, if you are significantly overweight, you are at greater risk for vitamin D deficiency, too (Holick, 2004). Which brings us to the following question: "Does your physician routinely screen for vitamin D deficiency?" Many do not. They may have not read my book **Mommy, Me, and Vitamin D**. Please, Mom, screen your physician for *this* unfortunate situation, and take the necessary steps. My book makes an excellent gift. You can give it to your doctor, to your daughter, to all your daughters and to all their friends, to your hair dresser, to your letter carrier, to your pastor, to your—the possibilities are endless!

Competitors and disruptors

The most common causes of maternal hypothyroxinemia are dietary iodine deficiency <u>and exposure to environmental antithyroid agents</u>.

Insufficient dietary iodine intake and a number of environmental antithyroid and goitrogenic agents can affect maternal thyroid function during pregnancy. **~Román, 2007, emphasis added**

In fact, a recent study points out that anti-thyroid environmental substances and pollutants can affect the thyroid function during pregnancy, increasing the risk of autism in the population. **~Berbel et al., 2009**

Environmental contaminants can disrupt thyroid hormone synthesis and inhibit iodine uptake and may thus induce maternal hypothyroxinemia. **~Hendrichs et al., 2013**

Bromide, used as a dough conditioner, is found in many breads. It competes with iodine at tissues, can inhibit thyroid hormone production, and can worsen iodine deficiency. Canada and some other countries have wisely banned its use. Avoid any food with ingredients such as potassium bromate, brominated vegetable oil, azodicarbonamide, etc. Enriched flower may contain bromide as an unlisted ingredient.

Fructose intake can create a copper deficiency, which in turn can decrease thyroid hormone production. Fluoride at concentrations found in drinking water has also been shown to damage thyroid tissue Other environmental toxins that depress thyroid gland and hormone function include PCBs, dioxins, DDT and its metabolites, aminotriazole, HCB, and phthalates.
~University of Kansas School of Integrative Medicine, 2013

If you want to fall asleep fast, or run the risk of slipping into a coma, try studying iodine competitors and thyroid hormone disruptors for any length of time. Four minutes is a length of time. Since I am all about reducing your risk of negative experiences, I will keep this section as short as possible. Here is what you need to know (try not to fall asleep).

We live in an environment of zillions of natural and man-made chemicals, some that interfere with the creation and utilization of thyroid hormone, while others block the uptake of iodine and increase the risk of iodine deficiency. Some are very prevalent in our environment and some can be found in common use in our society. Others are less common but can pose a threat to certain individuals who are regularly exposed. I will point out the biggies:

- **Tobacco smoke** (Román, 2007; Diamanti-Kandarakis et al, 2009). Danger! Danger! *"Decreased T4, increased TSH, and thyroid enlargement have been reported among women who smoke. Another study showed an association between cigarette smoking and decreased breast milk iodine concentration."* (Yarrington and Pearce, 2011)

- **Pollutants**, including pesticide and rocket fuel residues, in addition to chemicals used in manufacturing—particularly in the plastic and petrochemical industries—are considered thyroid hormone disruptors (Diamanti-Kandarakis et al, 2009). Apparently, there are over 150 industrial chemicals that reduce circulating levels of thyroid hormone (Diamanti-Kandarakis et al, 2009). Drinking water in coal- and shale-rich geographical regions can be contaminated with powerful antithyroid chemicals (Román, 2007).

- **Dietary components** found in soy products and in certain vegetables like broccoli, cauliflower, kale, kohlrabi, Brussels sprouts, rutabaga, cassava (inadequately soaked or cooked), millet, yams, sweet potatoes, sweet corn, bamboo shoots, and lima beans all have antithyroid and goitrogenic effects. (Román, 2007; Zimmermann, 2009). Bromide, added to breads, and added to some soft drinks and sports drinks (*Web*MD, 2013), can worsen iodine deficiency (University of Kansas School of Integrative Medicine, 2013). Soy products inhibit the uptake of iodine and decrease T3 and T4 availability (Román, 2007). Based on the ability of soy to block the uptake of iodine by the thyroid, soy-based formula has been reported to produce goiter in infants (Diamanti-Kandarakis et al, 2009).

- **Epoxy-lined food cans?** Yes, epoxy-lined food cans. Something as innocent as a can of vegetables can interfere with the thyroid hormone status of an individual. The offending chemical is called BPA. One group of investigators *"estimated human consumption of BPA from epoxy-lined food cans alone to be about 6.6 µg per person per day."* (Diamanti-Kandarakis et al, 2009) Recently, due to concerns about the harmful effects of BPA, baby bottles and sippy cups can no longer contain this chemical. (source: NYTimes.com, July 27, 2012)

- **Nitrates** act as a mild inhibitor of the uptake of iodine (Yarrington and Pearce, 2011). *"It [nitrate] is present in soil and ground water, and is found in virtually all crops,* *particularly root vegetables. Sodium nitrate is also used as a food preservative. The average daily adult intake of nitrate per day in the U.S. is 75–100 mg daily."* (Yarrington and Pearce, 2011)

- **Mercury.** Women have been advised to limit seafood to two servings per week while pregnant or nursing. The reason? It may be high in mercury. But why eat fish, say I, when you can get all the mercury that you don't need from your dentist. Dental amalgam "silver" fillings contain relevant amounts of this toxic substance. Why on earth is it still being used? *"During pregnancy, Takser et al. found a significant correlation between inorganic mercury levels in umbilical cord and lower maternal serum free thyroxin (T4) levels and concluded that even low levels of exposure to persistent environmental contaminants interfere with thyroid status during pregnancy."* (Román, 2007) Interestingly in one study, *"a related finding was the observed decrease in anti-thyroid antibodies in patients with autoimmune thyroiditis after removal of dental of dental amalgam fillings."* (Román, 2007) I'm not sure we should be doing this "dental amalgam thing," at least not during pregnancy, not when it represents a potential threat to our babies.

I am particularly concerned over bromide (and everything else mentioned above). They sneak bromide into our daily bread without even asking permission. It doesn't want to be evil, it just is. Several countries have wisely banned its use. It displaces iodine from its binding sites, preventing its uptake within the thyroid gland (University of Kansas School of

Integrative Medicine, 2013). The good news is that iodine supplementation reportedly increases the removal of bromide, bumping bromide off of binding sites and eliminating it via the urine (Abraham, 2003). Apparently, bromide is more of a threat if an individual's iodine status is low (University of Kansas School of Integrative Medicine, 2013).

It should also be noted that, in the past (before bromide came along), iodine was commonly used as a dough conditioner, nicely contributing to our daily intake of iodine. In fact, in the 1960s, if you purchased the right loaf of bread, one slice would net you 150 µg of iodine (Leung and Pearce, 2007). Two slices, and your daily requirements of iodine were covered. Unfortunately, potassium bromide seems to be here to stay (unless I have something to say about it). Get used to reading product labels! Stay as far away from bromide, in its many forms, as is reasonably possible, say I. Supplement adequately with iodine, say I.

In closing: If an individual's iodine or thyroid hormone status is marginal, relevant exposure to any one or all of these thyroid hormone disruptors could push someone over the edge. And as far as the food items mentioned above, just to be safe, eat them in moderation, and make sure you are receiving adequate iodine to compensate for their disruptive behaviors. Apparently, iodine sufficiency goes a long way to limit the impact of substances that block the uptake of iodine (Zimmermann, 2009).

He's worried. And he has a paper and a video.

Perhaps the best review of the environmental chemicals and dietary components that interfere with thyroid function or lower iodine levels is found in a paper written by Dr. Román in 2007. He also has a video. Search for:

Román GC 2007 Autism: Transient *In Utero* Hypothyroxinemia Related to Maternal Flavonoid Ingestion during Pregnancy and to Other Environmental Antithyroid Agents. Journal of Neurological Sciences 262:15–26

—Dr. Gustavo C. Roman. Autism Four Times Likelier When Mother's Thyroid Is Weakened. http://vimeo.com/71916860

Note: Dr. Román is worried about several environmental factors that interfere with the production of maternal thyroid hormone and decrease the availability of T4 for the developing fetus. Particularly at risk is the fetal brain. He presents compelling evidence that autism results, at least in part, from environmental and dietary exposures that interfere with thyroid hormone availability during gestation.

I'm worried, too. And I have a book (but no video)

Speaking of autism, maternal vitamin D deficiency has been identified as a risk factor for this devastating condition. Because I am alarmed when I find babies at risk of dying or living a life of compromise, I wrote a certain little book, entitled **Mommy, Me, and Vitamin D**. (I think I've mentioned this book before.) If you are vitamin D deficient during pregnancy—happens so easily—you are placing your pregnancy, your baby, at risk of some very bad things. As one research team states:

Vitamin D deficiency during pregnancy is the origin of a host of future perils for the child. Some of this damage done by maternal vitamin D deficiency becomes evident after many years. Therefore, prevention of vitamin D deficiency among pregnant women is essential. (Kaushal and Magon, 2013)

To find out what these "perils" are, read **Mommy, Me, and Vitamin D**. Someone is counting on you. This book can be ordered from my website:

—www.impactofvitamind.com

Chapter 4
The impact of iodine deficiency

*All degrees of iodine deficiency (**mild***: iodine intake of 50–99µ/day, ***moderate***: 20–49 µg/day, and ***severe***: 20 µg/day) **affect thyroid function of the mother and the neonate as well as the mental development of the child.** ~Delange, 2001, emphasis added

Iodine deficiency is the most devastating event in the developing brain in the fetus and neonate. Iodine is absolutely necessary on the myelination, neuronal differentiation, and formation of neural processes, synapto-genesis [creation of nerve connections], and neuronal migration by thyroid hormones throughout pregnancy and shortly after birth. ~Sarici et al., 2013, emphasis added

Iodine deficiency interferes severely with prenatal and post natal growth and neurologic development of individuals. It has condemned tens of millions of children to cretinism—characterized by mental and growth retardation, rigid spastic motor disorders, deaf mutism, and severe hypothyroidism—and hundreds of millions to milder degrees of mental and physical impairments. ~Hollowell and Hannon, 1997

Iodine deficiency may result in grave consequences for the whole population as iodine is the main component of thyroid hormones. This is why iodine deficiency in pregnancy may lead to goiter and hypothyroidism in women and, in consequence, to irreversible brain damage of the fetus. ~Matuszek et al., 2011

S o much of what we have discussed thus far has to do with iodine deficiency and its negative impact on the thyroid status of the expectant mother and her unborn baby. So much so, I thought I should devote an entire chapter to the impact of iodine deficiency. I did, and you are reading it now.

It takes about 200 micrograms of iodine per day to prevent pregnancy-associated goiter (Dunn and Delange, 2001). *"The clinical signal that iodine deficiency is severe is the prevalence of goiter . . . ."* (Hong and Paneth, 2008)

Recall, a goiter occurs when the thyroid is enlarging in order to extract (think, *desperately* extract) more iodine when iodine deficiency exists. *"In such settings, women enter pregnancy with some degree of subclinical hypothyroidism, which is then accentuated by the iodine and thyroidal demands of the pregnancy and fetus."* (Hong and Paneth, 2008) As the thyroid gland begins to respond to low iodine availability, and initiates the process of enlarging to form a goiter, *"the synthesis and secretion of thyroid hormones is altered. And switched toward a preferential use of the decreasing iodine supply to favor the secretion of T3 over T4."* (Morreale de Escobar et al., 2007) Under these circumstances, the mother's TSH may be normal, a sign that she is "euthyroid," but the developing baby will face a shortage of T4 (Morreale de Escobar et al., 2007).

It is the mother's response to low iodine availability that places her baby at risk for a negative outcome. As Mom is going about the business of building a bigger thyroid, Baby is going about the business of trying to develop normally—but will have to do so under the cloud of hypothyroidism. *"Under circumstances of sustained iodine deficiency, a shift in T3/T4 balance will occur in favor of T3."* (Verheesen and Schweitzer,

2008) Due to this "switch," Baby will face a shortage of T4. I sure hope things will turn out okay.

Iodine deficiency, like hypothyroxinemia, is deceptive. You don't feel it, and it is difficult to test for it in any meaningful way (Gronowski, 2012). Furthermore, in iodine deficiency thyroid hormone testing may be normal, particularly the TSH, giving the impression that there must be enough iodine around when this may or may not be the case.

A lack of iodine in the diet may result in the mother becoming deficient, and subsequently the fetus. **The mother and the fetus, however, respond differently to this situation, with the mother remaining euthroid and the fetus becoming hypothyroid.** (Skeaff, 2011)

See how deceptive this is! Things need careful consideration, not casual investigation or the absence thereof. Is there a pattern of living that suggests iodine deficiency? Does the patient in question avoid iodized salt? Is iodine absent or insufficient in her prenatal supplement? Does she drink certain citrus-flavored drinks, non-stop, such as citrus-flavored soft drinks or certain sports drinks containing bromide in the form of brominated vegetable oil? Does she live on bread, often loaded with bromide? Is she a vegetarian or a vegan (both diets known to be low in iodine and proportionally high in foods that block iodine uptake)? So many questions to ask. So much screening to do. And what does the lab work suggest? Is the $fT4$ level low? Has it ever been drawn? There is so much not being considered when we assume that we, as a people, are iodine sufficient and therefore our pregnant ladies and those of child-bearing years are iodine sufficient as well.

Even if iodized salt is regularly used and seafood is eaten a few times per week, that won't be enough to become iodine sufficient. *"Using iodized salt and eating seafood 2–3 days per week a woman's daily iodine intake would be in the order of 100–150 µg per day, approximately half the amount recently recommended during pregnancy and lactation."* (Berbel et al., 2009) And many do not use iodized salt at all. And many do not eat seafood at all. And along comes pregnancy, and iodine sufficiency, if it does indeed exist, is changed into something else, something sinister called iodine deficiency. *"Iodized salt consumption, promoted for years in areas that are now classified as free of iodine deficiency may not be sufficient for pregnant women."* (Berbel et al., 2009) *"Therefore, it is recommended that pregnant and lactating women receive daily iodine supplements (i.e., 200 µg of iodine) from the onset of pregnancy or earlier."* (Román, 2007) However, even *this* many not be enough. It may take as much as 250–300 µg of iodine per day to meet the needs that arise during pregnancy (Morreale de Escobar et al., 2007). It is imperative that our ladies who make babies become iodine sufficient.

Furthermore, although early maternal hypo-thyroxinemia can be important in fetal brain development, iodine deficiency may be even worse than isolated maternal hypothyroxinemia/hypothyroidism because of the additional problem of fetal hypothyroidism due to the lack of iodine availability for fetal thyroid hormone synthesis. (Negro et al., 2011)

The problem with iodine deficiency is that it damages and destroys babies. If severe, it causes fetal death. If less severe, it still causes fetal death. If severe, it causes cretinism, and mental retardation. If less severe—even mild to moderate iodine deficiency—it gives rise to any number of neurological abnormalities (e.g., autism) and a blunting of the intellect

(Román, 2007; Berbel et al., 2009). **Iodine deficiency in the mother leads to T4 deficiency for the developing fetus. The fetus now has a disease called hypothyroidism, and birth defects and unfavorable outcomes can follow.** Iodine deficiency is the cause of immense damage. And mommies and daddies fail to get what is promised: a healthy baby, arriving on time and ready to lead a happy, healthy life. Few know what is behind a good share of this devastation. I do. And I cannot remain silent.

> In the United States, <u>a seven-fold increase</u> in the frequency of moderate iodine deficiency among pregnant women has occurred since the 1970s, along with a four-fold increase in the frequency of moderate iodine deficiency in the total population, coincident with a greater than 50% decline in urinary iodine excretion, along with subclinical signs of thyroid deficiency. (Román, 2007, emphasis added)

I'm worried. So much trouble ahead! With respect to iodine sufficiency in the USA, I think we, indeed, have a little myth on our hands. Let's do a little myth-busting in the next chapter.

Iodine, soooooo important!

Here is a great video clip on the importance of iodine nutrition and supplementation during pregnancy:

—Iodine and Pregnancy
   www.youtube.com/watch?v=O8eHJLAOD1Y

The American Thyroid Association has a nice printout on iodine deficiency. I want you to have it. It provides the latest recommendations for iodine intake during pregnancy. Find and read the following:

   —Iodine Deficiency
      www.thyroid.org/patients/brochures/IodineDeficiency_
      brochure.pdf

Chapter 5
The myth of iodine sufficiency

In order for pregnant women to produce enough thyroid hormones to meet both her own and her baby's requirements, a 50% increase in iodine intake is recommended. A lack of iodine in the diet may result in the mother becoming deficient, and subsequently the fetus. ~**Skeaff, 2011**

A recent published study revealed that as many as 25% of pregnant women in the United States have iodine intakes that are less than half those recommended during pregnancy. ~**Morreale de Escobar et al., 2004**

As iodine status is based on median urinary iodine excretion, even in countries regarded as iodine sufficient, <u>a considerable part of the population may be iodine deficient.</u> ~**Verheesen and Schweitzer, 2008, emphasis added**

In the U.S., there is a higher prevalence of mild iodine deficiency in the pregnant population compared to the general population. ~**Yarrington and Peirce, 2011, emphasis added**

Iodine supplementation is necessary in geographical regions where dietary intake is not adequate, such as the USA, New Zealand and Australia. ~**Stagnaro-Green and Pearce, 2012**

I t is generally assumed that we, as a nation (USA), are iodine sufficient. This is a myth. This myth is a tragedy.

It all started back in the 1920s, a time when we "conquered" iodine deficiency (or so we thought) with the fortification of salt with iodine. Before this period of time, goiter was endemic in the Great Lakes, Appalachian, and the Northwestern regions of the United States (Lockwood, 2013). *"In addition to large goiters, affected women had pregnancy complications and their offspring had severe developmental delays."* (Lockwood, 2013) At this point in our history, we knew the cause of goiter and we knew its cure. And we conquered. Goiter due to iodine deficiency—that is, big ugly goiter due to iodine deficiency—soon became uncommon. Today, based upon this success, many individuals are under the impression that iodine deficiency is a thing of the past . . . and so we sleep, and a myth is perpetuated—all stemming from the success of salt iodization vs. goiter, regarded as one of our *"nation's greatest public health success*es." (Lockwood 2013) But it was not iodized salt alone that came to our rescue.

As the 20th Century progressed, other things came along that helped maintain a reasonable level of iodine sufficiency in our population. We all know that cows are dirty, so we used iodine preparations to clean the dirty cow before we milked the dirty cow. Due to this practice, iodine in significant amounts showed up in our milk supply (Leung and Pearce, 2007). We also began to use iodine in food processing, particularly as a dough conditioner, making our daily bread yet another good source of dietary iodine (Leung and Pearce, 2007). Then along came "progress."

Today, our dirty cows are often cleaned with some diabolical cleaning agent that does not contain iodine, and there have been restrictions placed on the amount of iodine that can be added to cattle feeds, further limiting iodine availability to our population and our dirty cows (Pearce et al., 2004). And if that weren't enough, we pulled this stunt: We removed iodine from our daily bread, replacing it with, of all things, bromide as a dough conditioner. As we have previously discussed, bromide is evil, it displaces iodine from binding sites and cannot be incorporated into the manufacture of thyroid hormone—effectively lowering an individual's iodine and thyroid hormone status. To make matters worse, we somehow arrived at the notion that salt is certainly out to kill us all. Accordingly, we were educated to reduce salt consumption and many of us did. As a result, overall, our iodine intake has declined. I apologize on behalf of our society.

> The current push to reduce salt intake in order to lower risks of hypertension and cardiovascular disease as well as increasing intake of noniodized salt from processed foods and sea salts or kosher salts have measurably reduced US dietary iodine intake. (Lockwood, 1013)

So, what does this progressive reduction in iodine availability look like? It looks like this: *"As a consequence of these cumulative trends, **US iodine stores dropped by 50% from 1970s levels** . . . ."* (Lockwood, 2013, emphasis added) Were you aware of this? Are you alarmed? (You should be.)

Is it beginning to sound a little like we have an iodine sufficiency myth on our hands? It certainly sounds like it to me! But a statistic is just a statistic—except this one damages, and this one kills. "Oh, but we have prenatal vitamins!" (Did I actually hear you say this, or am I hearing voices again?) Surprisingly, **only 28%** of prenatal vitamins contain iodine! (Lockwood, 2013) (*What planet am I living on?!!*) I'm beginning to think that we truly are asleep at the wheel. We are definitely not listening to the warnings. *Iodine deficiency kills babies!* It damages them, too.

This is the point in the chapter where you say, "Hum, perhaps we are in a little trouble due to iodine deficiency here in the good ol' USA." Oh, you want trouble? *I'll show you trouble!*

You could be one of these kind of people: You could be a healthy young lady, one who is trendy and therefore uses sea salt instead of iodized salt. You are lean, which, of course, is good, but you are also a runner. A big marathon is coming up, so you will be training a lot, and training means sweat. Sweating removes iodine from the body at a very fast pace (Smyth and Duntas, 2005). I hope you don't plan to get pregnant any time soon! You may not have what it takes to meet the increasing demand for iodine that pregnancy brings. Recall, when a pregnant woman is iodine deficient, she may not be able to supply enough T4 to meet the developmental needs of the one living inside. Abnormal outcomes and fetal demise may occur. And if this healthy runner is you, you are trouble! And you have not a clue that, should you be pregnant, you could be placing your baby at great risk due to iodine deficiency . . . by being healthy and being fit! Oh! Speaking of sweat: Let's hope you do not take a sauna on a regular basis (sauna, of course, equals more sweating and more iodine loss). And I just had this unsettling thought: I sure hope you are not a vegan.

Oh no! So now you are telling me that you are a vegan! Now we're talking trouble! This dietary practice is okay in many respects, but it clearly limits one's intake of iodine (Leung et al., 2011). No fish, no eggs, no meat—all good sources of iodine. I see trouble ahead.

The lesson in all of this is: Just because iodine is available, it doesn't mean everyone will be getting (or keeping) enough (Verheesen and Schweitzer, 2008). Many factors are in play.

The presence of iodized salt in an iodine-deficient community does not always protect reproductive outcome. Usual medical practice decreases salt intake during pregnancy, precisely the time when the mother needs more iodine, so iodized salt alone may not provide enough for her child's proper development. (Dunn and Delange, 2001)

And then along comes pregnancy, a time when everything changes. Should your level of iodine have been sufficient, up until this moment in time, it may not be enough now to meet the increasing demands of pregnancy.

Pregnant women need more iodine than this baseline requirement, to cover the iodine needs of the developing fetus and to compensate for increased renal [kidney] losses. Renal clearance of iodine increases during pregnancy. (Dunn and Delange, 2001)

Yes, there is a myth out there, and a dangerous one indeed. It is the belief that because, overall, our population has conquered iodine deficiency in the past—and overall we seem to be getting enough iodine as a population, enough so that big ugly goiters are rare—a problem is not hanging over the head of those who are or may become pregnant at a moment's notice. Indeed, a recent publication (2004) reported that *"7.6% of pregnant women in the USA are still affected by moderate to severe iodine deficiency."* (Hollowell and Haddow, 2007, emphasis added) We are not sounding any alarms (well, I am), there is no sense of urgency here! Oh, that's right! What we need are more studies before we start paying more attention to the ones we already have, studies that clearly warn us of the dangers. (I am being a little cynical in that last statement, can't you tell? Sorry.) Is *anyone* paying attention to the fact that in recent years our iodine consumption is 50% less than 30 or 40 years ago? And is *anyone* paying attention to the fact that the need for iodine increases by 50% during pregnancy? I am. And I'm trying my best to get your attention. Am I succeeding?

How to choose a prenatal

Choosing a prenatal vitamin is not as straight forward as one might expect. Here, I will share with you a few thoughts on the subject, for what it's worth.

Most prenatal formulas contain folic acid—a vitamin proven to prevent a variety of birth defects—but some formulas do not. What, then, is a mother to do?

It seems most reasonable to take extra folate in the form of folic acid, pre-pregnancy and in the first month or so following conception. As the pregnancy progresses, the benefits of folic acid supplementation are less clear and may or may not be advised (Charles et al., 2005). Discuss these issues with your physician. Then there is iodine.

A good share of the prenatal vitamins available today do not contain this most important ingredient, and some contain only teeny tiny amounts, probably by accident. For a supplement, this must be very embarrassing—iodine may be the most important ingredient a prenatal can contain, **period!** Of course, you would expect me to hold this opinion.

You already know of the importance of iodine. It should be in adequate supply. A prenatal with iodine is probably in order. So, how much iodine should you take? And what are the side effects to watch for? Both are issues to discuss with your physician. More than likely, a supplement containing at least 150 to 200 mcg (µg) will be recommended. And then there is B12.

Another nutrient that should be included in relevant amounts in a prenatal vitamin is vitamin B12. According to WebMD, *"Women with B12 deficiency in early pregnancy were up to five times more likely to have a child with a neural tube defect, such as spina bifida, compared to women with high levels of B12."* (WebMD, 2009, emphasis added) Many ladies are deficient in this vitamin, a nutrient derived almost exclusively from foods of animal origin—and the small amount of B12 in a prenatal may not fulfill your need, especially if you are vegetarian or vegan. You may need a higher dose than can be found in a prenatal; you may need to take a sublingual B12 so that it is more effectively absorbed; or, you may need a B12 shot, periodically, in order aggressively manage a major deficiency. I suggest that pregnant ladies (vegetarian, vegan, and others with certain medical conditions that place them at risk) be tested for B12 deficiency and be supplemented aggressively, should a deficiency exist. In one study, approximately 1 in 20 pregnant women were found to be deficient in B12, and at a time in their pregnancy when neural tube defects occur (Thompson et al., 2009). So, B12 deficiency during pregnancy is not all that rare. And it may be evil. Let's just say it is evil.

When choosing a prenatal, there is one more thing to keep in mind: Typically, a prenatal vitamin will contain iron as an ingredient. But do you need extra iron? Many assume that you do. Due to this assumption, iron finds its way into, perhaps, a majority of prenatal vitamins, yet few are aware of the dangers.

Here is the problem with iron: You need it, but you don't need too much of it. An excess of iron on board can lead to gestational diabetes and its associated, serious complications (Scholl 2005; Helin et al., 2012). Indeed, one study found a two- to threefold increase in gestational diabetes in those who supplemented with iron (Bo et al., 2009; Helin et al., 2012). Ask your physician about this issue, too. Other problems can also occur during pregnancy if you take iron and you don't need iron, including creating potentially harmful deficiencies in copper and zinc, (Ziaei et al., 2007; Hwang et al., 2013). Listen up! *"Iron supplementation for pregnant women should be individualized according to their iron status."* (Hwang et al., 2013)

It may be that, when it comes to prenatal vitamins, one may need to supplement the supplement! For example, with an otherwise suitable prenatal, one without iodine or low in iodine, you may need to take the missing amount in a separate tablet. Potassium iodide is generally recommended. Get your physician excited about iodine sufficiency then sort things out. Correct, *thoughtful*, prenatal supplementation is so important. Lousy prenatal supplementation may not achieve the goal in mind.

Want a suggestion?

While I have no intention here to endorse any product or mention any company name, I will offer you a suggestion or two with respect to the choosing of a good prenatal vitamin.

I found an excellent (my opinion) prenatal formula online by searching, using the words *prenatal vitamins without iron*. I won't mention the company name, GNC. And I won't mention the product name, *Prenatal Formula Without Iron*. I won't even mention the low suggested retail price of $9.99. The reason I won't mention any of this is because I don't want to endorse any product or mention any company name. However, if I *were* to tell you about this prenatal supplement, I would probably mention that it contains the recommended amount of iodine, folic acid, and B12 (although more B12 may be needed for certain individuals), and the great thing is, this formula does not contain iron, an ingredient that may be problematic if not needed. But I probably won't mention any of this because I do not want to mention any company names or endorse any products.

And while I am not mentioning any company names or endorsing any products, I won't mention the name *Nordic Naturals*. And the product name I don't have in mind is probably not *Prenatal DHA*. Since DHA, a nutrient that supports normal neurodevelopment, and is not typically found in a prenatal, supplementing with DHA may be strongly recommended. Your physician is the one who should make the call. One word of caution: **Do not**, unless instructed to do so, add another prenatal vitamin to the one you are already taking to fix the problem of a missing ingredient or two. By doing so, you could get too much vitamin A if both supplements contain this particular nutrient. Back to DHA. Based on my review of the literature, supplementation with DHA seems to be a wise choice to make. Ask the doc! I think I've not said enough, so I guess we should move on.

Note: I wrote the above skit, truly, not to endorse any product, but to get you thinking and help point you in the right direction. I, personally, went shopping, visiting several stores looking for the best in prenatal vitamins, to see what a shopper might face. I was <u>greatly</u> disappointed with what is generally available, and quickly realized that the reader could use a little help in knowing where to locate a prenatal that contains enough iodine to meet current recommendations. Furthermore, if one is fortunate enough to find a prenatal with a satisfactory amount of iodine, it will probably contain iron, an ingredient not always appropriate, according to the literature.

Clearly, choosing a prenatal vitamin is not just something to do. Choosing a prenatal is a _very_ important decision to make. My hope is, by offering a suggestion on where to start your search, and offering a suggestion or two on what to look for, you will be able find a prenatal vitamin that is most appropriate for your needs. Online shopping may be the best place to start. But whatever you do, your physician should be involved in any decisions you make. Print out and take product information with you when you go to have this discussion. But first, at least get started on _something_ that contains the recommended amount of folic acid, **ASAP!** Why? To be most effective in preventing neural tube defects, folic acid needs to be taken very early in the pregnancy and, if possible, before pregnancy begins. Get started on folic acid when you first suspect that you are pregnant or when considering pregnancy, per the current recommendation, then refine your prenatal vitamin options with your physician. (And, of course, try to find a prenatal vitamin with the recommended amount of iodine.) A prenatal can make all the difference in the world, but it will need to be the right one to meet your needs and it will need to be taken in a timely manner.

Chapter 6
You will be missed

Every effort *must be made to detect and prevent early maternal hypothyroxinemia to prevent neurodevelopmental defects, which may include an increased chance of lower IQ and a higher risk of cerebral palsy.* **~Negro et al., 2006, emphasis added**

The availability of THs (thyroid hormones) is critical for brain development. A growing body of clinical and experimental evidence indicates that ***even slight decreases in serum [blood] levels of THs can have significant consequences on brain development.*** **~Nucera, 2010**

The ***implications are staggering*** *when one considers that there is a significant increase in intrauterine deaths, spontaneous abortions, premature births and pre-eclampsia in women with gestational subclinical hypothyroidism.*

In the infant, <u>*major malformations*</u> *and loss of IQ could be prevented by early diagnosis and treatment of the mother [with hypothyroidism].* **~Mitchell and Klein, 2004, emphasis added**

It is <u>*mandatory*</u> *for doctors taking care of pregnant women with thyroid disease to have a thorough knowledge of the evolution of the normal thyroid function during pregnancy as well as during treatment of thyroid dysfunction in order to avoid such unfortunate and unnecessary cases.* **~Feldt-Rasmussen et al., 2011, emphasis added**

*In conclusion, **our study confirms that a case-finding strategy
for screening thyroid function would miss about 81.6% pregnant
women with hypothyroidism and 80.4% pregnant women with
hyperthyroidism.*** ~Wang et al., 2011, emphasis added

I t should be abundantly clear, by now, that women should be
routinely (and carefully) screened for thyroid hormone
abnormalities, both before (if possible) and as early as possible
in a pregnancy. It has also been recommended that <u>routine</u>
screening also be performed sometime later in the pregnancy
just in case things change and thyroid issues develop . . .
unexpectedly (Moleti et al., 2009). Certainly, screening for
thyroid hormone problems would be helpful at the beginning or
mid-point of each trimester in order to catch thyroid
abnormalities as the pregnancy progresses. And by screening, I
don't mean just checking a TSH. And I don't mean just checking
a TSH, with a $fT4$ level performed on the blood sample only if
the TSH is above normal. This sort of screening is a guarantee
that you will be missed . . . if you have hypothyroxinemia. But
you won't be alone. Hypothyroxinemia is hardly rare: *"While
the incidence of hypothyroidism in pregnant women is around
2.5%, hypothyroxinemia is much more prevalent, **up to 30%,
and it is usually due to <u>mild</u> iodine deficiency.***" (Bernal, 2014,
emphasis added) Recall reading this?

**Maternal hypothyroxinemia is an asymptomatic
condition for the mother, but it is <u>extremely harmful</u> for
the fetus.** Because the fetus's thyroid is still too immature
to synthesize sufficient T3 and T4, the fetus relies on the
maternal thyroid hormone for its optimal brain
development. (Opazo et al., 2008, emphasis added)

In hypothyroxinemia the TSH is normal, so a normal TSH means nothing here. And did someone say *"extremely harmful?"*

And I see another major problem: Thyroid autoimmunity will also be missed if the TSH is the only test run. And, of course, *nothing* will be found if testing is simply not performed.

> The negative influence of thyroid autoimmunity, even without hormonal thyroid dysfunction, on miscarriage and preterm delivery has been well established in the last decade and adds more arguments to take action so as to prevent these thyroid-related threats to pregnant women and newborns. (Vila et al., 2014)

In this book, I shared with you the risks of unidentified and untreated thyroid-related problems, problems which occur (rather frequently) during pregnancy; you paid close attention, and you were alarmed (I hope). At this point in time, I doubt if you are in the mood for not being screened. And I'm hoping you are not in the mood for just a screening TSH, along with the happy thought that, if normal, all is well from a thyroid hormone standpoint. There are babies at risk here! They must be found at all costs. It takes more than *nothing* and more than a TSH to identify all who are at risk. *"Every effort must be made."* (Negro et al., 2006) *"Unfortunately, not every effort is being made."* (The Author, 2014)

Of course I am always glad when a TSH is drawn, but, as I shared with you before, a TSH is not the final word on anything. That being said, a TSH is a very valuable test. It will help the physician find those with unsuspected hypothyroidism as well as those who have unidentified subclinical hypothyroidism, conditions that would otherwise go unnoticed. It may also prompt the physician to test for antithyroid antibodies—good call! But, like I say, if the TSH is normal and no further testing is performed, hypothyroxinemia, should it exist, will be missed. And thyroid autoimmunity, should it exist, will also be missed. Babies will be missed, and some will be lost, never to be found. (You're shedding a tear right now, aren't you?)

I am particularly concerned about hypothyroxinemia; I've shared with you the dangers. But I am very concerned about antithyroid antibodies; there are many good reasons to make the effort to detect their presence. *"Elevated maternal thyroid autoantibodies during pregnancy are linked to infertility, miscarriage, and neurodevelopmental defects such as in cognitive function."* (Wasserman et al., 2007, emphasis added) Furthermore, as the pregnancy progresses, antithyroid antibodies can lead to the development of hypothyroidism or hypothyroxinemia in the mother (Feldt-Rasmussen et al., 2011; Hendrichs et al., 2010). And later, antithyroid antibodies, having crossed the placenta before birth, can, in rare instances, create a period of prolonged hypothyroidism in the new little arrival (Sreedharan et al., 2012)—all unnoticed because someone decided that we need only screen those at high risk, and someone else decided to follow that advice.

So now, are you beginning see why I hold such strong feelings in opposition to the practice of screening only those considered to be at high risk for thyroid disorders? *"In the infant, **major malformations** and loss of IQ could be prevented by early treatment of the mother."* (Mitchell and Klein, 2004, emphasis added).

Unless action is taken to test every pregnant woman as early as possible (or even before conception), society will continue to pay a heavy price in the number of damaged offspring. (Mitchell and Klein, 2004)

Thyroid dysfunction in the first 20 wk of pregnancy may result in fetal loss and dysplasia [abnormal development] and some congenital malformations. (Su et al., 2011)

Targeted case finding

It is controversial whether screening programs for thyroid disorders in pregnancy should be universal or targeted case-finding. **~Jiskra et al., 2011**

Our study confirms that a case-finding strategy for screening thyroid function would miss about 81.6% pregnant women with hypothyroidism and 80.4% pregnant women with hyperthyroidism. **~Wang et al., 2011**

Consistently, over half of women with thyroid laboratory abnormalities would be missed if only high-risk women were examined. **~Jiskra et al., 2011**

Vaidya et al. revealed the limitation of targeted screening, which overlooked one third of pregnant women with hypo-thyroidism. Likewise, Horacek et al. recently reported the benefit of universal screening which detected twice as many thyroid disorders as targeted high-risk case finding. **~Lepoutre et al., 2012**

Boy I wish targeted case finding was good news! And it is for those lucky enough to benefit from this approach. Targeted case finding certainly helps identify many who are at an elevated risk of thyroid dysfunction during pregnancy by confirming what is suspected, based on the patient's health history or the presence of certain signs and symptoms.

Under targeted case finding, this is how you are screened: You show up at the doctor's office. You wait. You wait. And you wait. Then, when your name is called, they get your weight. Then you wait. Eventually, it's your turn to be evaluated. You are asked several questions while the physician looks over your medical records (if you have any). The physician, at this time, will want to know: **1)** if you have a family history of thyroid disease; **2)** if you have a personal history of thyroid disease including antithyroid antibodies, goiter, or thyroid surgery; **3)** if you have experienced any of the classical signs of hypothyroidism (*"although only 30% of cases usually show clinical symptoms"*); **4)** if you have any autoimmune diseases, particularly type 1 diabetes; **5)** if you are over 30 years of age (pre elderly); **6)** if you are morbidly obese; if you have experienced infertility, have had repeated pregnancy loss, or have delivered a premature baby in the past; and **7)** if you have received treatment with lithium, amiodarone, or have recently received an iodine contrast media during an imaging procedure. (source: Vila et al., 2014) There are other determinations made during the universal screening encounter, to be sure. But you will be missed (your baby will be missed) if the answer is "no" to all of the above areas of inquiry, and accordingly you are not tested to make sure that you do not have a thyroid hormone issue that lies hidden from view. Consider the following—read it carefully:

> The current Endocrine Society Clinical Practice Guideline recommends that targeted screening should be performed at the first prenatal visit, or at the diagnosis of pregnancy, on only those pregnant women who are in risk groups. However, Vaidya et al. showed that this approach results in missing as many as 30% of cases of both overt and subclinical hypothyroidism. Moreover, Horacek et al. confirmed that screening detects twice as many thyroid disorders in early pregnancy than targeted high-risk case-finding. (Matuszek et al., 2011)

Targeted case finding, in effect, means we will have more learning-disabled kids than we should, we will have more cerebral palsy kids than we should, we will have more autistic children than we should, we will have more babies that will never be held by their mommies due to pregnancy loss . . . than we should. It's very hard for me to be in favor of targeted case finding. We should be doing something else.

When the potential adverse outcomes are so significant and the tools to diagnose and intervene are easily accessible, however, leaving maternal thyroid disease underdiagnosed, even in one third of pregnant women, is no longer acceptable. (Brent, 2007)

Universal screening

In view of the potential for serious adverse events associated with maternal thyroid disease, and the apparent benefits of treatment, many have recommended routine thyroid function screening in pregnancy. **~Brent, 2007**

*Rates of pregnancy-related events were reduced by nearly 40% after detection and treatment. This effect was large enough that **approximately 40 low-risk women would require screening (and intervention) to prevent a single adverse pregnancy outcome**.* ~Alexander, 2010, emphasis added

In the USA, a regional screening laboratory charges approximately $5 to measure TSH and T4, supply the filter paper and report the results. Since approximately 1:1000 newborns is at risk of brain damage due to maternal <u>subclinical hypothyroidism</u>, the cost of identifying a child at risk is approximately $5000. Clearly, this is a cost-effective approach.

We believe that if screening of all pregnant women is implemented, the mother, the infant and society will all benefit. **~Mitchell and Klein, 2004, emphasis added**

My! This *is* good news. Finding 1 baby at risk out of 40 in those who are believed to be in the low-risk category is good news indeed (Alexander, 2010). *Wonderful!* And so many at-risk babies can be found. Thousands of babies! **Thousands!** This is the power of universal screening. This approach, universal screening, <u>will</u> save babies.

> From the second trimester onward, the major adverse obstetrical outcome associated with raised TSH in the general population is an increased rate of fetal death. If thyroid replacement treatment avoided this problem this would be another reason to consider population screening. (Allan et al., 2000)

"Not me! Not my baby!" It's beginning to sound like you are developing a little attitude here! I would! This is serious business, the detection of thyroid hormone abnormalities in <u>everyone</u> who is pregnant (or likely to become pregnant)—and not just in those who fall within the high risk category. That is why you will be hearing from a highly-respected authority on things that really matter, Dr. Roberto Negro. I will let him end this chapter for me.

> Personally, I stand in favor of universal screening for thyroid disease at the beginning of pregnancy. We have to consider that in Western countries the mean age of first pregnancy is 25–30 years, and a recent report showed that in women older than 25 years more than 15% have thyroid abnormalities. Furthermore, everyone agrees that it is necessary to treat overt thyroid dysfunction, and in particular overt hypothyroidism. A recent paper published by Dosiou and coworkers clearly shows that universal screening is cost-effective not only compared with no screening, but also compared with screening only women at high risk for thyroid dysfunction. Notably, in this analysis

the authors assumed that women with any degree of hypothyroidism receive treatment, but only women with overt hypothyroidism benefit from treatment. My personal opinion is that, above all in countries with high-quality healthcare systems, a 25–30-year-old woman at her first pregnancy has the right to know if she is hypothyroid, at risk of developing hypothyroidism, or at risk of developing a postpartum thyroiditis. TSH and TPO antibodies should be the first test used to screen a woman for thyroid dysfunction. A TSH concentration >2.5 mIU/L in the first trimester, and >3.0 mIU/L in the second and third trimester, should be considered as pathologic. (Gronowski, 2012, interviewing Dr. Robert Negro)

All in favor say "Aye"

> *Many professional associations of endocrinologists have taken varying views, with evidenced-based review panels concluding that there is insufficient evidence to recommend universal screening, while other expert groups advocate [universal] screening.* ~**Matuszek et al., 2011**

To me, universal screening is a no-brainer. A missed child? Missed children on a grand scale? Statistically, 88,000 new babies in the US are born each year to mothers with an elevated TSH (Dosiou et al., 2008). And we can find at-risk babies so easily, just by testing!!! What on earth are we waiting for? We are waiting for this: We are waiting for more organizations to climb on board. Currently, unless there has been a very recent change, only the National Academy of Clinical Biochemistry is in favor of universal screening (Matuszek et al., 2011). However, a press release, dated October 16, 2013, indicated that 74% of thyroid specialists surveyed at the 2012 annual meeting of the American Thyroid Association (ATA) were in favor of universal screening (American Thyroid Association, 2013). On the other hand, surprisingly (to me), the American College of Obstetricians and Gynecologists, the American Association of Clinical Endocrinologists, as well as the ATA, still remain reluctant to endorse universal screening (Vila et al., 2014). Indeed, *"the American College of Obstetricians and Gynecologists has recommended against screening all pregnant women for hypothyroidism and against treating subclinical hypothyroidism."* (American Association of Clinical Chemistry, 2012, emphasis added) So, once again, it's smart people vs. smart people, but I'm a common-sense kinda guy. Universal screening just makes good common sense. I would not want my baby to be missed, possibly lost, possibly damaged, due in part to the commonly-held belief that universal screening is not justified. *Are you kidding me?!!*

Not far enough

There is universal screening, then there is universal screening . . . on steroids! *This* is what I am in favor of. Let me explain: It is one thing to screen for thyroid hormone problems before and at the beginning of pregnancy. However, as pregnancy progresses, with the added stress and strain on preexisting iodine stores and impaired thyroidal performance, problems do pop up, unexpectedly—problems that will go unnoticed unless testing is repeated. *"Indeed, pregnancy represents a challenge for the maternal thyroid, due to a progressive increase in hormone demand that can only be met by a very marked augmentation in hormone output."* (Moleti et al., 2009) So, in my opinion, universal screening is not just for before pregnancy and not just for at the beginning of pregnancy, it is for the entire pregnancy, with a low threshold for testing at any given point in time. And, of course, it includes close attention to the iodine status of the mother along the way. Is she taking a prenatal with iodine every morning? Is she throwing up her prenatal every morning? Is she smoking? Does she have a lifestyle practice (or several) that restricts iodine intake or increases iodine loss? If she is just squeaking by in the iodine department, the new baby may run very low on this vital element within weeks of birth, and become hypothyroid during a key period of neurological development (Soldin et al., 2013; Akinci et al., 2006).

You Will be Missed, the movie

I have located an excellent video clip regarding targeted case finding vs. universal screening . . . just for you. I want you to watch it. You don't have to, but you need to. Go to *The Doctor's Channel* online and, in the search box provided, type in "Case finding approach." Click on:

—**Case finding approach misses most cases of thyroid disease during pregnancy**

Chapter 7
Spare the children

The greatest impact of iodine deficiency on cognitive and neurological function occurs during gestation and early infancy.
~Hollowell et al., 1998

Thyroid hormones are essential for normal brain development . . . beginning from the intrauterine period <u>and extending through 1–2 years of age</u>. During pregnancy, both maternal and fetal thyroid hormones are required for normal fetal brain development. **~Akinci et al., 2006, emphasis added**

*Epidemiological studies have indicated that <u>even a marginally low</u> thyroxin [T4] level in a pregnant woman may give rise to reduction in cognitive function of the offspring. Thus, **even <u>minor</u> changes in the thyroid homeostasis may affect neurological development**.* **~Boas et al., 2012, emphasis added**

Infants younger than 1 year are at high risk for iodine deficiency because their requirements per kilogram body weight for iodine and thyroid hormones are higher than at any other time in the lifecycle. Even in countries where most other age groups are iodine sufficient, infants can have insufficient intakes.
~Bouhouch et al., 2013

This is a very important chapter. Children are very important people. And so many are placed at such great risk. They are at risk of abnormal development (damage), both before birth and after, not by things that are rare, but by things that are commonplace. Iodine deficiency and hypothyroxinemia are not exactly rare.

A recent published study revealed that as many as **25%** of pregnant women in the United States have iodine intakes that are <u>less than half</u> those recommended during pregnancy. (Morreale de Escobar et al., 2004 emphasis added)

While the incidence of hypothyroidism in pregnant women is around 2.5%, hypothyroxinemia is much more prevalent, **up to 30%**, and it is usually due to <u>mild</u> iodine deficiency. (Bernal, 2014, emphasis added)

Here, in this chapter, we will take a look at some of the damage inflicted upon our precious little children, one child at a time—damage caused by iodine deficiency and low T4 in ladies who make babies. Some of this damage has a name, like autism, cerebral palsy, and developmental delay. But regardless of the name, there would be less autism, less cerebral palsy, and less developmental delay if we were to make <u>certain</u> that our pregnant ladies, and those of child-bearing years, were iodine sufficient . . . and that <u>any</u> abnormality in thyroid function were promptly identified and properly addressed, one lady at a time. Is *this* too much to ask? By now you *must* be convinced that universal screening is necessary and long overdue. Babies are at risk here! This chapter should drive the message home.

One thing to keep in mind: Before one can become a new-born baby or even a child, he or she may have to survive the effects of even "mild" thyroid hormone insufficiency in Mom. And it may not be all that easy. *"Even mild maternal thyroid dysfunction has been reported to be associated with spontaneous abortion and fetal death."* (Su et al, 2011, paraphrased) Astonishingly, depending on the method of detection upwards of **70%** of pregnancies are lost, a large percentage within the first few weeks following conception (Haymart, 2010). And those who make it out alive, what will their fate be?

Autism

Maternal hypothyroidism causes pregnancy complications, including postpartum hemorrhage, placental abruption, and preterm labor; some of these are risk factors for autism.
~**Román et al., 2013**

In fact, a recent study points out that anti-thyroid environmental substances and pollutants can affect the thyroid function during pregnancy, increasing the risk of autism in the population. ~**Berbel et al., 2009**

Of related interest is the finding that a family history of autoimmune thyroiditis doubled the risk of autism. ~**Román, 2007**

Animal models confirm that the first half of pregnancy may constitute a sensitive period in which maternal hypothyroxinemia alters neurogenesis and causes neuronal migration errors in the developing fetal brain. ~**Hendricks et al., 2013**

Autism is a complex neurodevelopmental disorder that affects a child's social development, including the ability to communicate and associate normally with others. It may or may not have an effect on the intelligence of the child. Autism can give rise to unusual behaviors, repetitive behaviors, and odd preoccupations. It can be mild, or it can be devastating.

In autism, something is wrong with the brain. It did not develop properly. "What *ever* could have gone wrong?" you ask. I will tell you.

In the brain, during its development, there are highways of scaffolding that somehow emerge from out of nowhere for the purpose of guiding stem cells as they migrate to their target location in the brain. (Román, 2013; Bernal, 2014) However, when fetal T4 availability is low, this migration is impaired, yielding a brain that is improperly assembled—with certain cells not located in the correct place and, therefore, unavailable to be called upon to perform specialized tasks (Bernal, 2014; Palha and Goodman, 2005; Hendrichs et al., 2013). Additionally, the cells that have managed to arrive at the right location, will need to change or differentiate into their final form. Cellular differentiation is also impaired when thyroid hormone levels are low (Hendrichs et al, 2013). Thus, silently, a disaster is in the making—eventually yielding a brain that is not a good one, a brain characterized by structural compromise and altered performance (Bernal, 2014).

Autism is, indeed, a disaster, and certainly worthy of concerted efforts aimed at its prevention. But it is doubtful that we will stem the tide of the autism epidemic we are experiencing unless we start paying more attention to the iodine and thyroid hormone status of mothers during pregnancy (and before), as well as paying more attention to the iodine and thyroid status the new little arrival. Consider this:

> Iodine deficiency is the most devastating event in the developing brain in the fetus and neonate. Iodine is absolutely necessary on the myelination, neuronal differentiation, and formation of neural processes, synapto-genesis [creation of nerve connections], and neuronal migration by thyroid hormones throughout pregnancy and shortly after birth. (Sarici et al., 2013, emphasis added)

A couple of years ago, I had a neighbor with autism. He was a handsome, normal-looking teenager in every way, but could not speak. According to his very loving and supportive mother, his favorite thing in life was to go outside, stand on the back porch, and make hooting sounds (repeatedly, every few minutes). He was severely autistic, but, thankfully, others with this disorder are less afflicted. But afflicted they are. And autism, in any form, is not at all what you or your child want to experience. However, should it occur, your child will not be alone. The numbers are quite alarming and on the rise.

In 2006, when I stated to pay attention, 1 in 150 children in the USA were reported to have autism. And I thought *this* stat was disturbing! Three years later, when I began the research phase of this book in earnest, the autism rate had increased to 1 in 88 children. Now, in 2014, approximately 1 in 68 children will become autistic. Hearts will be broken. Lives will be broken. And so few are aware that something as simple as iodine deficiency, and/or low T4 levels in Mom during pregnancy, may, in many cases, be to blame.   Careful universal screening for iodine deficiency and thyroid hormone dysfunction—as well as screening for environmental disruptors that limit iodine uptake and thyroid hormone production—has the power to prevent disasters in the making, one child at a time.   Of course, screening will be useless unless corrective action is taken.

Cerebral palsy (CP)

Thyroid deficiency in utero during critical periods of brain development causes mental retardation, psychomotor delay, and deafness. It is also associated with other neurodevelopmental outcomes such as cerebral palsy.   **~Ares et al., 1997**

Nelson and Ellenberg report that children of women who were **hypothyroxinemic or hyperthyroxinemic** *both before or during pregnancy may have poor fine motor coordination, varying* *degrees of mental retardation, specific signs of cerebral palsy (including spasticity, tone abnormalities, and hemiparesis), and a* **20-fold increase** *of risk for later cerebral palsy.* **~Hollowell and Hannon, 1997, emphasis added**

Scientists have linked low levels of a thyroid hormone in premature infants to the development of disabling cerebral palsy. They examined more than 400 premature infants screened for blood levels of the hormone thyroxin during the first week of life. They found that **infants with low levels of thyroxin at birth had a 3- to 4-fold increase** *in the incidence of cerebral palsy at age 2.* **~National Institute of Neurological Disorders and Stroke, 1996, emphasis added**

Every effort must be made to detect and prevent early maternal hypothyroxinemia to prevent neurodevelopmental defects, which may include an increased chance of lower IQ and a higher risk of cerebral palsy. **~Negro et al., 2006**

Cerebral palsy is a condition wherein the brain, due to injury or malformation, is unable to properly control muscles. Loss of use follows and painful muscle spasticity can result. Cerebral palsy can cripple the body, and it can cripple the mind. It may be mild or it may be devastating—requiring total care of paralyzed individual . . . for life. The leading risk factor for cerebral palsy is prematurity. And the statistics are quite alarming.

The prevalence of cerebral palsy at age 3 years is 44 per 1000 infants born at <27 weeks, 21 per 1000 of those born between 28 and 30 weeks, and 0.6 per 1000 for those delivered at term. (Yoon et al., 2003)

The above statistics should come as no surprise, as prematurity is an open invitation for many unfavorable events to transpire, events that have the capacity to inflict severe damage on a developing brain. Surprisingly, the risk of cerebral palsy in premature infants with severe hypothyroxinemia is **"4.4** *to 17.6 times that of infants with normal thyroxine (T4) concentrations."* (Reuss et al., 1996, emphasis added) "Why?" (I knew you would ask.)

With prematurity, the baby's little thyroid gland may not be able to compensate for the abrupt loss of maternal T4 (Negro et al., 2006). Hypothyroidism would then follow the untimely birth, and would occur during a critical time for brain development—hence an increased risk for brain damage, hence an increased risk for cerebral palsy, hence an increased risk for unimaginable heartache and devastation. Additionally, with prematurity, a life-and-death struggle may ensue, with serious illness hampering the ability of the new little one to maintain adequate thyroid hormone levels.

However, the risk of cerebral palsy is also elevated when the mother, therefore the baby, is hypothyroxinemic during the course of a term pregnancy, no prematurity required (Zoeller and Rovet, 2004). Thus, we see developing babies without enough T4 on board, for any reason, are at increased risk for this most unfortunate outcome.

Cerebral palsy has many other causes, to be sure, but hypothyroxinemia in Mom is certainly one risk factor that we can do something about. Correcting hypothyroxinemia may even prevent the prematurity that gives further rise to the hypothyroxinemia that an untimely birth so often brings. Hypothyroxinemia can be prevented, can be detected, and can be successfully treated (typically with iodine supplementation—see Männistö, 2013). This is why universal screening is *so* important. It can identify those who are at risk for hypo-thyroxinemia as well as other thyroid disorders that have the power to harm the most vulnerable in our midst.

"Several studies have related disorders of thyroid function in mother or infant to motor disability or CP in the

child, and to cognitive limitation or deafness." (Nelson, 2009)

How many cases of cerebral palsy can be prevented by close attention to the iodine/thyroid status in Mom? That's a good question. It could be quite high. But saving one baby from cerebral palsy would be reason enough for us to be <u>diligent</u> in finding those who are iodine deficient as well as those who have thyroid hormone abnormalities.

Of course, in order to reduce the chance of acquiring cerebral palsy, the premature baby will need to be watched very carefully with regard to his or her thyroid status, with a diligent search conducted for any opportunity to correct thyroid hormone issues that arise. And arise they will. <u>Low T4 levels will be found in 35–50% of premature infants, and prematurity occurs in about 12% of all births</u> (Berbel et al., 2010). Unfortunately, dealing with low T4 in the preemie is not all that straight forward, and treatment may actually be inappropriate, at least during the initial days and weeks postpartum (more later).

Because cerebral palsy can be so devastating, considerable nursing care is often required, with no end in sight. Accordingly, the average lifetime cost to the family of an individual with cerebral palsy is estimated to be on the order of $921,000 (source: CerebralPalsy.Org). And we're worried about spending a few bucks on thyroid screening! Tell me again, what planet are we living on?

I made this section a little longer than intended, but I am very upset at cerebral palsy right now. I take care of these patients from time to time in my nursing practice. And it tears my heart out. Some of this is *so* preventable. (Sigh!) Let's end this section with the following:

Despite advances in medical care, cerebral palsy remains a significant health problem. The number of people affected by cerebral palsy has increased over time. This may be because more and more premature infants are surviving. In the United States, about 2 to 3 children per 1,000 have cerebral palsy. As many as 1,000,000 people of all ages are affected. Cerebral palsy affects both sexes and all ethnic and socioeconomic groups. (Alvarez, 2014)

Efforts to detect and prevent maternal hypothyroxinemia in early pregnancy appear fully justified. Indeed, neurodevelopment defects, including an increased probability of cerebral palsy, may be 150 times more frequent than those resulting from untreated congenital hypothyroidism. (Calvo et al., 2002, emphasis added)

Attention deficit hyperactivity disorder (ADHD)

ADHD is a developmental disorder involving difficulties with sustained attention, distractibility, poor impulse control, and hyperactivity or inability to regulate activity level to situational demands. **~Vermiglio et al., 2004**

The most important finding, and totally unexpected, was that **70%** *of the offspring of mothers, with mild iododeficiency [iodine deficiency] had ADHD, while it is not diagnosed in offspring of mothers in a control area with iodo [iodine] insufficiency.* **~Lopez, 2012, emphasis added**

Thyroid antibody positivity has been associated with . . . attention problems and aggressive behavior, in children. **~Männistö, 2013**

So, what is ADHD? The quick answer? For a parent and for a teacher, it is a *big* challenge. For the child with ADHD, it makes for a rough go in life.

All children with ADHD may struggle with low frustration tolerance and trouble following rules. Often they are "poor sports" in games, and they may seem intrusive or bossy in their play. As a result, children with ADHD face social challenges because their peers may perceive them as immature and annoying. They may be taunted by peers or tricked into getting into trouble with adults. Whereas older adolescents are able to describe their difficulties due to ADHD, children frequently have trouble identifying their underlying difficulties. Instead, children with ADHD are often only aware that they get into trouble more often than their peers, leading to self-doubt and low self-esteem. (Massachusetts General Hospital, 2010)

Surprisingly, little attention is given to the role low T4 and low iodine availability plays in the development of ADHD, not at all the attention that it should receive. You may have never heard any of the following before I came into your life:

There is mounting evidence that <u>even mild</u> maternal thyroid under-function may be associated with impaired fetal brain development.

Furthermore, a 10-yr follow-up of the progeny of mildly-deficient women carried out by our research group showed a high proportion (70%) of children with attention deficit and hyperactivity disorders and defective IQ scores among those born to mothers who had experienced hypothyroxinemia (but not hypothyroidism) during early gestation.

It is worth mentioning that in our series of pregnant women, isolated hypothyroxinemia was, by far, the most frequent sign of thyroid insufficiency. (Moleti et al., 2008, emphasis added)

The association between low T4 during gestation and ADHD is strong indeed. We should take heed.

Before we move on, let's take another look at some of the challenges ADHD creates. This birth defect damages how well a life can be lived.

Attention Deficit/Hyperactivity Disorder, or **ADHD**, is a medical condition that makes it hard for people to regulate their attention, organize themselves, and control their impulses. For some people with the hyperactivity component of ADHD, keeping quiet, staying seated, or stopping all body movements is nearly impossible. While everyone may have occasional moments of daydreaming, fidgeting, or forgetfulness, someone with ADHD experiences these difficulties often, in multiple settings, such as home and school, over a period of at least 6 months.

ADHD may significantly affect a child's life by impairing academic activities, peer relationships, and home life. Estimates of the prevalence of ADHD among children range from 3 to 12 percent. The tendency to develop ADHD involves complex genetic and environmental factors. Although the disorder occurs more frequently in boys than in girls, its prevalence in girls is greater than previously thought. (Massachusetts General Hospital, 2010)

Learning, behavior, ability, and delay

As mild to moderate iodine deficiency is still the most widespread cause of maternal hypothyroxinemia, the birth of many children with learning disabilities may be prevented by advising women to take iodine supplements as soon as pregnancy starts, or earlier if possible, in order to ensure that their requirements for iodine are met. **~Morreale de Escobar et al., 2007**

Moreover, delayed iodine supplementation of hypo-thyroxinemic mothers during early pregnancy is associated with a higher risk of neurobehavioral delay. **~Hendricks et al., 2013**

Any maternal iodine deficiency results in a range of intellectual, motor, and hearing deficits in offspring. This loss in intellectual capacity limits educational achievement of populations and the economic prowess of nations.

Through the past millennia, the loss of human intellectual, physical, and social potential caused by iodine deficiency has been enormous. **~Maberly et al., 2003, emphasis added**

Velasco et al., found that children of mothers supplemented with 300 µg of iodine in the first trimester had higher psycho-motor development scores than children from mothers who did not start supplementation until the last month of pregnancy. **~Skeaff, 2011**

Given that 2.2% of pregnant women have an elevated TSH, out of about 4 000 000 pregnancies that occur annually in the US as many as 88 000 infants are at risk of low IQ. **~Dosiou et al., 2008**

Since prematurity is a risk factor for so many adverse outcomes—and since preemies after birth are typically low in T4—it should come as no surprise that approximately half of those born prematurely, will exhibit mild cognitive impairment (Zoeller and Rovet, 2004). *"Particularly affected are their visuospatial and fine motor skills, selective attention and memory abilities, math competency and contrast sensitivity."* (Zoeller and Rovet, 2004). And as always, things can go from bad to worse.

> Studies evaluating the consequence of hypothyroxin-emia of prematurity have reported an increased incidence of cerebral palsy, reduced intelligence and poor psychomotor abilities in children whose TH [thyroid hormone] levels were low at birth. (Zoeller and Rovet, 2004)

Aside from the challenge of prematurity, even if the baby arrives on time, I see trouble ahead.

> Women who are unable to increase their production of T4 early in pregnancy would constitute a population at risk for neurological disabilities in their children.

> As a mild to moderate ID [iodine deficiency] is still the most widespread cause of maternal hypothyroxinemia in Western societies, the birth of many children with learning disabilities may be prevented by advising women to take iodine supplements as soon as pregnancy starts, or earlier if possible. (Morreale de Escobar et al., 2007)

All things considered, is sounds like we <u>can</u> do something about the tragedy of developmental delay. We can start by doing something about the tragedy of iodine deficiency in ladies who make babies . . . and do so without delay.

> Deficiency of iodine, an essential component of thyroid hormones, determines thyroid hormone plasma levels. Clinical studies of iodine supplementation provide good evidence for the importance of this micronutrient. Delayed iodine supplementation of hypothyroxinemic mothers

during pregnancy increases the risk of neurodevelopmental delay in children. Moreover, thyroid peroxidase antibodies and autoimmunity can cause hypothyroxinemia; pregnant women with positive antibodies are more prone to develop hypothyroxinemia. (Hendrichs et al., 2010)

Insufficient iodine levels during pregnancy and the immediate postpartum period result in neurologic and psychological defects in children. (Leung et al., 2011)

Birth defects

Birth defects affect 1 in 33 babies.   ~**Lemacks et al., 2013**

*The **implications are staggering** when one considers that there is a significant increase in intrauterine deaths, spontaneous abortions, premature births and pre-eclampsia in women with gestational subclinical hypothyroidism.*

In the infant, <u>major malformations</u> and loss of IQ could be prevented by early diagnosis and treatment of the mother [who has hypothyroidism].   ~**Mitchell and Klein, 2004, emphasis added**

Babies born to women with overactive or underactive thyroid also were at increased risk of a variety of other anomalies, including cleft lip or palate, or extra fingers.   ~**John's Hopkins Medicine, 2002**

It has been already demonstrated that <u>both overt and subclinical</u> hypothyroidism during pregnancy are associated with obstetrical complications. Maternal complications include anemia, postpartum hemorrhage, cardiac dysfunction, preeclampsia, and placental abruption; fetal complications include fetal distress, premature birth, and/or low birth weight, <u>congenital malformations</u>, and fetal/perinatal death.   ~**Negro et al., 2006, emphasis added**

Due to thyroid hormone insufficiency imposed on the developing baby during fetal development, an opportunity is created for a variety of structural defects to occur. Recall, thyroid hormone orchestrates genetic events. And, of course, genes make body parts. So when thyroid hormone availability is insufficient during gestation, particularly early gestation, the formation of structures, parts, and "things" that are so very useful and necessary to have, may be altered. Some birth defects are noticeable, some are not. All are unwanted. And we should do all we can to reduce the risks. Again, I have something in mind. Certainly, by paying close attention the iodine and thyroid hormone status of our pregnant ladies and those of child-bearing years, I believe we could put a dent in the alarming incidence of birth defects. *1 in 33! OMG!*

During gestation, under-treated and unidentified hypo-thyroidism is an open invitation for trouble. Even subclinical hypothyroidism, a condition where T4 levels are normal (but often on the low side of normal), can lead to birth defects (Negro et al., 2006). But this does not need to be. A portion of the birth defects we see can be prevented with careful, complete—not reluctant or minimal—thyroid hormone screening.

> Our study confirms that a case-finding strategy for screening thyroid function would miss about 81.6% pregnant women with hypothyroidism and 80.4% pregnant women with hyperthyroidism. (Wang et al., 2011)

We need to identify _all_ pregnant women who are at risk, not only those who seem to be at risk. And so many are at great risk! Wouldn't it be nice to take a bite out of this 1 in 33 statistic? We can, but first we will need to start paying more attention to the iodine and thyroid hormone status of those who are pregnant and those who may become pregnant at a moment's notice.

Babies born to women with untreated hypothyroidism due to Hashimoto's disease may have a higher risk of birth defects than do babies born to healthy mothers. Doctors have long known that these children are more prone to intellectual and developmental problems. There may be a link between hypothyroid pregnancies and birth defects, such as cleft palate. A connection also exists between hypothyroid pregnancies and heart, brain and kidney problems in infants. If you're planning to get pregnant or if you're in early pregnancy, be sure to have your thyroid level checked. (MayoClinic, 1998-2011)

Why boys more than girls?

There is apparently a 4 to 1 boys over girls-ratio with autism and ADHD. Why? The obvious place to look is the effect various hormones have on the developing brain, particularly the effects of testosterone vs. estrogen. But has the following been factored in? And this may be important! Boys ordinarily pee out more iodine than girls (Leung and Pearce, 2007). This means that, in the setting of low iodine intake (or disruption—remember soy-based formula?) during the initial newborn and infancy period, less iodine will be available to complete the neurodevelopment that begins during gestation and continues in infancy. Consider this:

Infants younger than 1 year are at high risk for iodine deficiency because their requirements per kilogram body weight for iodine and thyroid hormones are higher than at any other time in the lifecycle. Even in countries were most other age groups are iodine sufficient, infants can have insufficient intakes. (Bouhouch et al., 2013)

Given that boys pee out more iodine than girls, given that infants have a greater need for iodine than anyone else on the planet, and given that infants are at high-risk for iodine deficiency; therefore, for any given iodine intake, a boy, generally, will have a lower iodine status than a girl. Hence, a boy will be more at risk for autism and ADHD. This is my take on the issue, for what it's worth.

What can be done about autoimmunity?

It may be possible to reduce the intensity of an autoimmune attack directed against the thyroid gland by taking or making enough vitamin D to be become vitamin D sufficient. This is something you should be doing anyway. Forget that measly little 400 IU of vitamin D in your prenatal. It is *"woefully inadequate."* (Hollis and Wagner, 2004) You need thousands, not hundreds, of IUs of vitamin D per day to become sufficient during pregnancy, according to the experts. Of course, you would know this if you had purchased and read my book *Mommy, Me, and Vitamin D*. (Shameless plug, I know).

Vitamin D modifies immune responses, and studies suggest that it may lessen the severity of the attack by antibodies against the thyroid gland (Shin et al., 2014). Vitamin D supplementation may even lower antithyroid antibody titers (Shin et al., 2014). A lower antithyroid antibody titer means less risk for an unfavorable outcome for the one who is developing inside.

Chapter 8
Recommendations

A 50% increase in iodine intake is recommend in order for pregnant women to produce enough thyroid hormones to meet fetal requirements. A lack of iodine in the diet may result in the mother becoming deficient, and subsequently the fetus.
~Skeaff, 2011

Hypothyroidism should be corrected before the initiation of pregnancy, replacement dosage should be augmented early in pregnancy, and euthyroidim should be maintained throughout.
~Ozdemir et al., 2013

The above two recommendations seem simple enough, but there are rules, exceptions, precautions, and contra-indications for all to consider. In this chapter, we will ask the experts to help us out so we do things right. But first—and this is important!—*please,* **act only under the advice and supervision of a medical professional**. Mistakes can be made if you go out on your own. For example, if you are iodine deficient, replacement with *"more than adequate"* or excessive amounts of iodine may, under certain circumstances lead to hypothyroidism, subclinical hypothyroidism, or thyroid autoimmunity, even hyperthyroidism (Teng et al., 2011; Pearce et al., 2013). Of course, never adjust your dosage of thyroid medication on your own. **Don't make me repeat this again!** Now, let's see what suggestions the experts have to offer us in order to make this iodine/thyroid hormone business work to our advantage. As we continue, remember why we are going to the trouble of learning all of this. We are out to prevent birth defects and negative outcomes.

Iodine supplementation issues

Recall from an earlier discussion, it takes 200 *m*cg/day of iodine to prevent pregnancy-associated goiter (Dunn and Delange, 2001). Therefore,

> A 50% increase in iodine intake is recommend in order for pregnant women to produce enough thyroid hormones to meet fetal requirements. (Skeaff, 2011)

What does a 50% increase look like? It may look like a total iodine intake, from all sources, of 350 mcg/day, perhaps more (Delange, 2004; Klubo-Gwiezdzinska et al., 2011). Ask your physician for his or her recommendation. Even before pregnancy, an increase in iodine intake is strongly recommended (Ogilvy-Stuart, 2002). A prenatal vitamin, one containing 150 mcg of iodine, may do the trick. However . . .

In order to supplement with iodine wisely, choose a formulation that is more standardized and reliable, as found in a potassium iodide supplement or in a prenatal vitamin containing this form of iodine. It may be prudent to avoid iodine derived from kelp or seaweed. *"Kelp and seaweed-based products, because of unacceptable variability in their iodine content, should be avoided."* (Zimmerman and Delange, 2004) So, now you are telling me that you have been advised to supplement with iodine. This comes as *great* news! However, finding the right prenatal may be a problem. *"Only 51% of the adult multivitamin formulations on the U.S. market contain iodine (generally 150 µg iodine daily)."* (Leung and Pearce, 2007) So, don't assume that a prenatal will contain iodine. If it's not on the label, it won't be in the product. Shop wisely, Mom, and with purpose. Look for the iodine. And make sure it is not from kelp.

> Currently 69% of prescription and 25% of non-prescription prenatal U.S. multivitamins contain iodine, many of which do not contain the labeled amount, especially when kelp is the iodine source. (Leung et al., 2011)

Iodine supplementation is not without risk, particularly if taken in excess. Be aware that **chronic high iodine intake may precipitate hypothyroidism or stimulate autoimmunity against the thyroid gland** (Teng et al., 2011). Therefore, to do things right, supplement with iodine in a recommended amount and under the watchful care of a physician. And please don't overdo it. More is not always better.

Warning! If your prenatal contains 150 mcg [µg] of iodine per tablet, and your physician advises you to take 300 mcg of iodine per day, **do not**, I repeat, **do not** take an extra prenatal or two per day to achieve the recommended amount of iodine, you may get too much vitamin A.

With respect to vitamin A, *"taking too much vitamin A during pregnancy can cause birth defects. Don't take more than 5,000 IUs (international units) of vitamin A per day."* (March of Dimes, 2009) But consuming excess vitamin A is not the only concern, should you take an extra prenatal vitamin or two per day. You could also be receiving too much iron. Unless you have iron deficiency anemia, it may not be safe to take any, let alone extra supplemental iron during pregnancy (Ziaei et al., 2007).

Keep the following in mind, too: Selenium plays a role in thyroid hormone metabolism, and selenium deficiency can lead to hypothyroidism (Morreale de Escobar et al., 2007). *"Selenium supplementation during pregnancy and in the post partum period also reduces thyroid inflammatory activity and the incidence of post partum thyroid dysfunction."* (Wang et al., 2011) However, in the context of both iodine and selenium deficiency, *"selenium supplementation may aggravate hypothyroidism . . . and should not be undertaken without concomitant iodine supplementation in an iodine-and-selenium-deficient population."* (Vanderpas et al., 1993) Be careful out there! As with iodine, supplement with selenium only under medical supervision.

In closing, even though there are some problems associated with iodine supplementation, keep the following in mind:

> The benefits of correcting iodine deficiency far outweigh the risks of supplementation as long as supplementation is not excessive. (Yarrington and Pearce, 2011)

T4 replacement recommendations

> *Many women with pre-existing hypothyroidism are diagnosed and treated with supplemental T4, but the majority of these women tend to be under-treated because their T4 doses are not increased to match the normal physiological demands for TH [thyroid hormone] during pregnancy.* **~Zoeller and Rovet, 2004**

Taking thyroid medication is not rocket science (well, maybe it is); however, there are a few important things to keep in mind so that mistakes are not made. We can start with this:

Only about 62–82% of all ingested levothyroxine [T4] is absorbed, with concurrent ingestion of food, caffeine and iron and calcium supplements decreasing the absorption further. (Männistö, 2013)

Accordingly, *"We advise the patients to take their LT$_4$ [levothyroxine/T4] tablet at least 30 minutes before breakfast to warrant the best therapeutic achievement."* (Yu et al., 2013) Dr. Männistö recommends a 60 minute interval between taking your thyroid medication and eating (Männistö, 2013).

It is also important that you <u>do not</u> take your prenatal vitamin at the same time you take your thyroid medication. *"Prenatal vitamin supplements commonly taken during pregnancy are rich in iron and calcium, both which inhibit thyroxin [T4] absorption."* (Ozdemir et al., 2013) Dr. Männistö insists that there should be a 4 to 6 hour gap between taking T4 and taking iron- and calcium-containing prenatal vitamins (Männistö, 2013). Therefore, it seems reasonable to take your thyroid medication first thing in the morning, say 30 to 60 minutes before breakfast, and then take your prenatal later, with lunch or with dinner.

This is important! Switching T4 preparations—i.e., substituting Synthyroid for Levothyroid—may affect how much T4 you receive. *"Indeed, in a survey to physicians treating patients with levothyroxine [T4], most reports of changes in thyroid function were after switching between levothyroxine products, often by the pharmacy without the physicians knowledge."* (Männistö, 2013) Bottom line: Stay on the medication as originally prescribed, and if a change is made, make sure your physician is the one making the change. And if a change has occurred, follow-up labs are definitely in order.

Another consideration: Anticipate an increase in the amount of thyroid hormone will be required once pregnancy has been confirmed. Don't forget to remind your physician of this (he or she is juggling so many things that this could be overlooked).

> Our data demonstrate that two additional T4 tablets per week, when instituted immediately upon confirmation of pregnancy, significantly reduce the risk of maternal hypothyroidism throughout pregnancy. (Yassa et al., 2010)

Even for those who are planning their pregnancy and, at the same time, are under treatment for hypothyroidism, an increase in the T4 dosage by one or two tablets per week has also been recommended (Yassa et al., 2010).

There is one more important thing to consider with respect to thyroid hormone supplementation before we move on. Based on personal experience, I can offer the following precaution: If you are taking a T3 preparation called Cytomel or, as in my case, a preparation called slow-release T3 (Liothyronine SR), if the dosage it too high this may drive your T4 level to an unacceptably low level. I actually had this experience, easily corrected by a simple dose adjustment. Recall, your baby needs only T4 from you, and the possibility exists that taking T3 in excess may lower your T4 levels to the hypothyroxinemic range. This may be harmful to your baby. Use caution when it comes to all T3 preparations, say I. Which brings me to this recommendation: Discuss all medications you are currently taking with your physician. Even over-the-counter meds used to control stomach acid can interfere with the absorption of your thyroid medication (Khandelwal, 2007). Even "natural remedies" under consideration or currently in use should be discussed.

Screening considerations

Since you live in a world where universal screening is, well, not universal, you may need to be a little assertive in order to become appropriately screened. I, personally, have found most physicians quite willing to order extra labs if the request seems reasonable. (Saving your baby seems reasonable.) So be an army of one! Request a complete thyroid work-up regardless of the standard of practice (and regardless of the cost to the insurance company or to you).

Screening programs can also be organized locally (as they are already established in several European hospitals nowadays). Finally, it is perhaps worth considering voluntary screening, whereby pregnant women would accept to pay the cost of measuring serum TSH, Free T4, and TPO-Ab [antibodies against the thyroid gland] in early pregnancy." (Glinoer and Smallridge, 2004, emphasis added)

What labs, then, should be drawn? We can ask Dr. Negro for his advice.

TSH and TPO antibodies should be the first test used to screen a woman for thyroid dysfunction. A TSH concentration >2.5 mIU/L in the first trimester, and >3.0 mIU/L in the second and third trimester, should be considered as pathologic. (Gronowski, 2012, interviewing Dr. Robert Negro)

Other experts recommend checking a *f*T4 level, and I couldn't agree more. I believe it is worth knowing if an individual has hypothyroxinemia, even before pregnancy. Why take the risk of not knowing, and why take the risk of not taking the steps necessary to effectively deal with this issue.

Most cases of maternal hypothyroxinemia are related to a relative iodine deficiency during pregnancy that can be so easily prevented, with minimal expense, without risk and with worldwide success. (Morreale de Escobar et al., 2004)

Screening is not just for before pregnancy nor reserved for the first prenatal visit, screening should also occur at intervals throughout the entire pregnancy. And what will the physician be looking for as the pregnancy progresses? He or she will be looking for an acceptable TSH or one that is abnormal.

The goal of LT_4 treatment is to normalize maternal TSH values within the trimester-specific pregnancy reference range (first trimester, 0.1–2.5 mIU/L; second trimester, 0.2–3.0 mIU/L; third trimester. 0.3–3.0 mIU/L). (Stagnaro-Green et al., 2011)

And, following corrective action taken for hypothyroidism,

It is recommended that maternal serum TSH concentrations should be measured approximately every 4 weeks during the first trimester and TSH should be checked at least once in the second half of gestation and at 6 weeks postpartum. (Soldin et al, 2013)

Finally, why wait for pregnancy to occur before being screened for thyroid dysfunction? Thyroid problems are so very common in women of child bearing age. And babies are so vulnerable. Just do it! Screening, followed by corrective action, will save babies. Screening, followed by corrective action, will prevent so much heartache and so much devastation. Due to the importance of these issues, perhaps more than one physician and perhaps more than one discipline should be involved should a major thyroid hormone issue arise. Well, let's see, *all* thyroid issues that occur during pregnancy are major.

> Pregnant women with thyroid disease should be diagnosed and the treatment managed preferably in multidisciplinary clinics, where obstetricians, endocrinologists, pediatricians and other healthcare professionals can jointly work together to reduce risks of adverse pregnancy and neonatal outcomes associated with thyroid disease. (Männistö, 2013)

Therapeutic considerations

Therapy for hypothyroidism during pregnancy is nearly universal, let's just say universal. Mom *will* get her T4! (I hope the dosage prescribed is sufficient enough and early enough to prevent fetal compromise, and is not taken at the same time as her prenatal.) If pregnancy seems likely, an increase in thyroid hormone by an extra tablet or two per week is recommended for those already under treatment for preexisting hypothyroidism (Yassa et al., 2010). Get your physician's approval first! As for the other thyroid disorders we have discussed, things are not so universal. However, for the Mom who is on a mission, should she have hypothyroxinemia, subclinical hypothyroidism, or thyroid autoimmunity, she should prepare herself to be assertive and <u>fearlessly</u> ask her physician to treat her thyroid abnormality according to what seems reasonable, as suggested in the research literature, even apart from what is considered the standard of practice. Be aware, it takes time for Medicine to change its ways and physicians to get up to speed on what's new, even on very important matters. And of course you are in no mood to wait until everyone climbs on board to receive the advanced care that may best protect your baby from harm. You want the <u>highest</u> level of care that Medicine can offer . . . now! (Well, maybe you don't, but you should.)

In the remainder of this chapter, I will assume that you have been properly screened and you have at least one of the following conditions.

Consider requesting therapy for the following:

For hypothyroxinemia:

The effective treatment for hypothyroxinemia, in most cases, may simply be iodine supplementation (Morreale de Escobar et al., 2004). For mom, the extra iodine on board will allow for the production of more T4. For the developing fetus, the extra iodine transferred from Mom may allow for an increase in fetal thyroid hormone production and may allow little Jimmy or little Susie (or whomever) to develop an iodine reserve from which to draw after birth. At some point in time, T4 supplementation for gestational hypothyroxinemia may be approved, but, for now, it is not currently recommended. We are waiting for the completion of a very important clinical trial (CATS trial) before a recommendation will be formally made whether to use or not use T4 to manage hypothyroxinemia during pregnancy (Stagnaro-Green et al., 2011).

For subclinical hypothyroidism:

Subclinical hypothyroidism during pregnancy may or may not be treated by your physician, depending on the guidelines that he or she follows (American Association of Clinical Chemistry, 2012; Stagnaro-Green and Pearce, 2012; Ghirri et al., 2013). But I know someone who believes we should treat it!

The well-respected Dr. Negro. *"I strongly support levothyroxine [T4] treatment in women with subclinical hypothyroidism before and during pregnancy."* (Gronowski, 2012, interviewing Dr. Negro) And, just so you know, he is not the only one trying to get others to climb on board.

Perhaps the warning of how serious subclinical hypothyroidism really is has not gone out as clearly as it should.

If you have subclinical hypothyroidism you may have a 3-fold increase in placental abruption and a 2-fold increase in preterm birth (Alexander, 2010) Furthermore, strong evidence exists that pregnant women with subclinical hypothyroidism have a "significantly increased risk" for severe preeclampsia (Wilson et al., 2012) Therefore, *"Careful follow-up of SCH [subclinical hypothyroidism] in pregnant women should be taken, and thyroid function should be tested every month until the end of pregnancy."* (Yu et al., 2013) Subclinical hypothyroidism is not benign. It is evil.

> Once the diagnosis of . . . [subclinical hypothyroidism] is made, the Guidelines of the Endocrine Society clearly recommend treatment with LT4. (Klubo-Gwiezdzinska et al., 2011)

For autoimmune thyroid disease:

Thyroid autoimmunity is not routinely screened for, but it should be! Request it. Don't let me down! (I am easily disappointed.) If your physician is not inclined to test or to treat, request a referral to a specialist, one who may be inclined to test and to treat. You can back up your request for testing and treatment of this disorder by sharing the following:

In a recent randomized interventional trial, miscarriage and preterm delivery rates were much lower in women with autoimmune thyroiditis given thyroxin [T4] (started at five to 10 weeks) throughout gestation to keep them euthyroid than in controls [those not receiving treatment]. The miscarriage rate was reduced by 75% and preterm delivery by 69% in women given thyroxine. (Glinoer and Abalovich, 2007

While you are all into sharing, share this, too:

Euthyroid women positive for the TPO Ab should be strongly considered for low-dose levothyroxine [T4] replacement (~50 µg daily) once pregnant. (Alexander, 2010)

Always keep in mind that thyroid autoimmunity during pregnancy is not benign. There are increased risks associated with this disorder.

Positive thyroid antibodies information may also be of interest, as their detection is a marker of a pregnancy with a higher risk than average, and therefore a closer follow-up could be performed. The safety of T4 treatment has also been confirmed in only one study, in which women with positive anti-thyroid antibodies with normal TSH received T4. (Vila et al., 2014)

For hyperthyroidism

Hyperthyroidism is typically treated with drugs that partially block the production thyroid hormone, thereby reducing an excess of circulating T3 and T4. If you receive a TSH test before or after pregnancy occurs, you will know whether you have hyperthyroidism. It's that easy. In this disorder, the TSH will be very low.

Hyperthyroidism during pregnancy typically requires treatment. However, treatment is not without risk. Therefore, it is better to receive effective treatment before becoming pregnant. However, if discovered early in the pregnancy, treatment with drugs used to block the synthesis of thyroid hormone can be carefully prescribed and things should turn out all right. Be sure to follow your physician's instructions to the letter. There is an ever-present risk of birth defects associated medications used to treat hyperthyroidism (Stagnaro-Green and Pearce, 2012). You will want to do things right, and, obviously, so will the physician.

> For best practice, in patients with overt hyper-
> thyroidism as a result of Grave's disease, the lowest
> possible dose of antithyroid drugs should be used during
> pregnancy with the goal of a serum free T4 level at, or just
> above, the trimester-specific upper limit of normal.
> (Stagnaro-Green and Pearce, 2012).

Drugs to avoid during pregnancy and nursing

The rule of thumb? All drugs should be avoided if possible during pregnancy and nursing, and this would include over-the-counter drugs, herbs, and natural remedies. Something as harmless as a cold remedy or an antacid can be inappropriate to use while you are pregnant. This is why *everything* should be discussed with your physician. When this is not feasible or the response time is not quick enough, you may want to check things out for yourself. There is a great little website that can help you screen for drugs that are safe and drugs that are unsafe to use during pregnancy and lactation. It is called *SafeBaby.com*. This website has a search box that will allow you to type in the name of the drug and with one click find out if it is safe to use during pregnancy. Great website!

Chapter 9
New and what to do

Iodine is critical for normal hormone synthesis and brain development during infancy, and <u>preterm infants are particularly vulnerable to the effects of both iodine deficiency and excess</u>.
~Belfort et al., 2012, emphasis added

Insufficient iodine levels during pregnancy and the immediate postpartum period result in neurologic and psychological defects in children.   **~Leung et al., 2011**

Prematurity is a tough spot to be in. The moment it begins, it is an abrupt end to a continuous supply of hydration, of nutrients and, of course, an abrupt end to the mother's transfer of thyroid hormone to the developing baby. With prematurity, Baby is not ready for this unfortunate turn of events, and will now have to take on the role of exclusively manufacturing his or her own thyroid hormone. Unfortunately, many babies who are born too early are just not up to the task. In this context, the risk of neurological damage is exceedingly great. "So, what can be done to minimize the risks?" I'm so proud of you. You are learning to ask the tough questions. Well, let's see. Perhaps we can make sure prematurity is not an abrupt end to an adequate supply of iodine.   This should help!   Let's start here. Accomplishing this could make all the difference in the world.

The challenge of prematurity

Over 12% of all births in the United States are preterm . . . and preterm infants are a particularly vulnerable population with respect to iodine nutrition. Preterm infants have lower iodine and thyroid hormone stores relative to full-term infants and require relatively more iodine than full-term infants and older children to maintain a positive iodine balance, so they are at risk for deficiency without adequate dietary intake. **~Belfort et al., 2012**

Thyroid hormone synthesis is critically dependent on an adequate prenatal and postnatal supply of iodine, which can paradoxically suppress T4 secretion when present in excess, especially in preterm infants and in the presence of iodine deficiency. **~Ozdemir et al., 2013**

Many are the challenges a premature baby faces, but iodine deficiency should not be one of them. Unfortunately, it so often is. While there may be a little iodine reserve available for the tiny little thyroid gland to work with, typically, this reserve will not last very long. Help will need to come from somewhere.

The recommended intake for the preterm infant is 30 µg/day (Feingold and Brown, 2010). If iodine is provided below this level, less thyroid hormone can be produced, which, of course, is problematic. So, there seems to be a pressing need to provide an adequate amount of iodine for the early new arrival. However, too much iodine can limit thyroid hormone production and create, or perpetuate, low T4 levels in the premature infant (Belfort et al., 2012; Ozdemir et al., 2013; Ghirri et al., 2014). So caution must be exercised. Of course all of this gives rise to a few rules to follow, rules that should be carefully considered.

The **first rule is maintain a positive iodine balance** in the premature baby. Accordingly, iodine supplementation is generally in order. This can be accomplished in a number of ways. If the preemie requires I.V. nutrition, it may be appropriate to add the recommended amount of iodine to the I.V. solution (Feingold and Brown, 2010; Belfort et al., 2012; Ghirri et al., 2014). Which brings us to this:

In the not too distant past—perhaps tragically—the need to add iodine to I.V. nutrition was not as much of a concern, as the iodine-based antiseptic solution previously in common use in the neonatal ICU became an unexpected source of iodine, perhaps too much iodine (oops!) (Feingold and Brown, 2010; Belfort et al., 2012; Ghirri et al., 2014). In fact, iodine-based cleansers probably harmed many preemies over the years, due to their suppressive effects on thyroid hormone production, leading to the creation or perpetuating of neonatal hypothyroidism. After this unintended consequence was identified, today the use of iodine-based cleansers is being actively discouraged in the neonatal ICU (Belfort et al., 2012; Ghirri et al., 2014). But this has given rise another problem: Now that we have entered an era wherein the use of iodine-based antiseptics is actively discouraged and limited, the amount of iodine in I.V. feeding solutions (if any) may now be too low to meet the needs of the preterm infant (Ibrahim et al., 2003; Ghirri et al., 2014). Mom, make sure this issue is addressed and the I.V. feeding solution (TPN) contains today's recommended amount of iodine, unless, for some reason, this is not advised. I'm sharing this information with you for a reason. I want you to know what to anticipate, and I want you to be able to ask all the right questions.

Be aware that, at some point in time, you may be asked to supply breast milk for your premature baby, in which case, you should also be encouraged to supplement adequately with iodine so your milk will be iodine sufficient (Ghirri et al., 2014). Human breast milk is so important, even for the preterm infant—so much so that donor milk from another lady (or a bunch of ladies pursuing an unusual career) is generally available. However, donor milk, without fortification, has been found to be unacceptably low in iodine (Belfort et al., 2012). But the breast milk from a baby's own mother is best, so if it is *you* who will be doing the honors, it is important that you be adequately supplemented with iodine. Therefore, your physician should be encouraging you to take iodine supplementation (and should be prescribing the appropriate amount to take). If this recommendation has not been made, you should bring it up as soon as possible—this could have been accidently overlooked. Some little someone is counting on you! And some little someone is counting on you not to smoke, even after birth. At least two studies have concluded that *"smoking decreases breast milk iodine concentrations."* (Leung et al., 2011)

Infant formulas are generally sufficient in iodine, but it doesn't hurt to ask if it is, just to be sure. If the formula is soy-based, raise a little fuss and insist that, if soy formula is absolutely necessary, it be one adequately fortified with iodine. (see Zimmermann, 2009)

Second rule: guard against iodine excess in the preterm infant. We have already discussed the fact that iodine excess can come from iodine-based antiseptic solutions used in the neonatal ICU. But excess iodine can also be transferred to the baby during birth if an iodine-based antiseptic is used as a prep for a cesarean delivery (McElduff et al., 2005). Another prep solution, one that is free of iodine, may be a better choice so as to avoid iodine-induced suppression of thyroid hormone production in the new arrival. And on a related note . . .

Douching with an iodine-based formulation while breast feeding is a big no-no. You will absorb at least some of the iodine found in the solution—perhaps too much—and you may transfer excessive amounts of the absorbed iodine to your baby and suppress his or her thyroid function (Feingold and Brown, 2010).

There is one final consideration that I need to bring to your attention before we move on. And it is this:

Now that you are breastfeeding, or otherwise providing your baby with your breast milk (I am making the assumption), there is another something important to consider. Although kelp is a good source of iodine, if eaten in excess or if kelp (a seaweed) is the origin of iodine in a vitamin/mineral supplement, the amount of iodine ingested, and passed via breast milk on to the nursing infant, may be excessive and may suppress Baby's thyroid hormone production, leading to, or perpetuating, neonatal hypothyroidism (Crawford et al., 2010). Fortunately, the ingestion of seaweed is not common in our culture, but in other cultures it is consumed to a considerable extent, hence the warning.

The **third rule is to consider often (ask repeatedly) if and when thyroid hormone supplementation is in order.** The preemie could have congenital hypothyroidism, a condition that may be missed in all the madness of prematurity—in which case, this condition will require some sort of thyroid hormone treatment, when circumstances allow. The earlier this condition is identified, the better. To detect congenital hypothyroidism and to look for opportunities for thyroid hormone treatment in general, frequent labs should be drawn to assess the thyroid hormone status of the preterm infant as things progress. Which brings us to the following question . . .

Can we safely supplement the preterm infant with thyroid hormone?

> *A common finding in preterm newborns is neonatal hypo-thyroxinemia. Neonatal hypothyroxinemia has been associated with cerebral palsy, mortality, morbidity, and intraventricular hemorrhage [bleeding in the brain]. Attempts have been made to replace T4 in premature infants with limited demonstrable results. In 2001 we recommended that hypothyroxinemia of the preterm infant should not be routinely treated in Neonatal Intensive Care Units, unless as part of an ongoing study.* ~**Simpser and Rapaport, 2010**

> *Our data suggest that thyroxin (T4) treatment of premature neonates should be attempted to compensate for the interruption of the maternal supply.* ~**Berbel et al., 2010**

Of course, the answer to the above question, whether we can supplement the preemie with thyroid hormone, is a yes, maybe. Although not part of the current the standard of practice, thyroid hormone supplementation of the preemie is apparently being done here and there, at least on a limited basis (Golombek et al., 2002). As a mother, one who wants the very best for her premature baby (and doesn't mind being a little assertive), perhaps the best approach is to request an endocrinology consult to help evaluate Baby's need for thyroid hormone therapy. I don't want to buck the trend, but your baby is very important to me, and I do not want an opportunity to slip through our fingers for an <u>appropriately-timed</u> intervention to occur. The more specialists involved, the better.

> Pregnant women with thyroid disease should be diagnosed and the treatment managed preferably in multidisciplinary clinics, where obstetricians, endocrinologists, pediatricians and other healthcare

professionals can jointly work together to reduce risks of adverse pregnancy and neonatal outcomes associated with thyroid disease. (Männistö, 2013)

It may be that thyroid hormone supplementation of the premature infant is appropriate at some point in time after birth, based on individual clinical judgment. Or, on the other hand, a conservative approach (stay the course) may be well-advised. Several great minds working together (yours included) may be best when it comes to sorting out the challenges of prematurity and knowing just what to consider next. And since we aware of the damage neonatal hypothyroidism can inflict on the preterm baby, we will want to do all we can to lessen the risk and resolve the problem.

And wouldn't you know, I have several studies to back up the feasibility of using thyroid hormone for preterm babies in order to squeak out a better clinical outcome.

One study found that low-dose T4 supplementation, given I.V., produced no adverse effect, and, unexpectedly, cut the mortality rate in half. (La Gamma et al., 2009) This is big! No, this is **Big!**

In another study, a one-time dose of T3, given I.V., was used in a study of very preterm babies—with the intent to mimic the T3 blood-level surge that typically occurs immediately after a normal, term birth (Cools et al., 2000). This treatment strategy was interpreted to be promising by the authors of the study, given that this strategy was found to sustain neonatal T3 levels for several weeks and *"without change in plasma T4 levels."* (Cools et al., 2000) Along the same line, an earlier study, using a single dose of T3 given to preterm infants 12 hours after birth, *"found increased plasma T3 levels for as long as 8 weeks with no clinical side-effects and <u>this therapy was associated with improved outcome.</u>"* (Zoeller and Rovet, 2004, emphasis added)

T3 therapy for the preemie does sound promising indeed, but as one study points out: *"The lack of any beneficial effect of T3 in our study may be explained by suppression of FT4 in the treatment group."* (Biswas et al., 2003). *A lowering of T4!—this* could be a problem. Are you beginning to see how tricky this thyroid-hormone business is in the preterm infant? Are you beginning to see why there is a justifiable reluctance to jump right in and treat the preterm baby with thyroid hormone? While many physicians would like to, great caution must be exercised. No one wants to make a mistake here.

I guess the bottom line in all of this is: When it comes to thyroid hormone supplementation for the preterm baby, ask the neonatologist involved to consult with an endocrinologist just to see if some form of thyroid hormone would be an appropriate course of action to take at some point in time.

> Some, but not all, forms of thyroid supplementation appears to reduce the incidence of poor neurodevelopment outcome in infants born at extreme prematurity. (Ng et al., 2008)

It never hurts to ask. And you never know when the standard of care will change and the green light will be given for thyroid hormone supplementation of the preterm bundle of joy.

I will close out this section with this:

> Our data suggest that thyroxin [T4] treatment of premature neonates should be attempted to compensate for the interruption of the maternal supply. (Berbel et al., 2010)

One more item to discuss, and another terrific gray box to go, then I'll bring this book to a close.

The risk of arriving right on time

Iodine deficiency is a major threat during pregnancy and early childhood as these periods are critical in the development of the neural system of the fetus and the child. ~**Ghirri et al., 2014**

Of course, the threat of iodine deficiency can extend beyond the womb. As we have discussed many times before, during gestation the baby should be developing an iodine reserve upon which to draw after birth. Unfortunately, if mom is iodine deficient, the baby, after birth, may not be able to manufacture enough thyroid hormone to meet his or her needs, at least on an ongoing basis. Furthermore, if Mom is nursing and is, at the same time, iodine deficient, the situation may not improve. Developmental issues can show up from out of nowhere, and some babies will eventually receive the diagnosis of autism, ADHD, or some other "something" you do not want you or your child to experience . . . forever.

Yes, iodine deficiency *is* risky business. On the other hand, adequate iodine intake during the pregnancy and while nursing will offer a degree of protection from the evils of which I speak.

Iodine supplementation for the infant and child

45% of the types of U.S. children's multivitamin formulations contain iodine, and importantly, none of the infant liquid multivitamin formulations marketed in the U.S. contain iodine. ~**Leung and Pearce, 2007**

Iodine is needed for the developing baby, both before and after birth. If the baby is nursing from an iodine-sufficient mother, or is bottle-fed with an iodine sufficient formula, this thing is covered. But what about the toddler and what about the older child? They need iodine too—brain still under construction! So what's a mother to do?

To answer this question, I looked for the nearest available expert, Fred Flintstone. Perhaps you have heard of him—I have been impressed with him for as long as I can remember. And, knowing just where to find him, I went shopping for children's vitamins to see what a mother might face. And to my surprise, Fred makes a tasty gummy that contains a respectable amount of iodine. And, as a bonus, I found one formula that does not contain iron. *This* was a good day for someone who doesn't want to mention the name of any company or product.

Quite frankly, I was surprised that Fred, being so old, was up to date and aware that most children do not need extra iron. Wisely, he kept it out of *Flintstones Gummies Complete* (suggested retail, $9.69). (Since I do not want to mention any company names or products here, I'm not sure how any of this slipped in.) "No iron in a multivitamin?" You may be surprised to hear this. But excess iron in children is not without danger.

> Iron can be toxic in children who have normal levels of iron, so you should not give iron supplements to a child without a doctor's supervision. (University of Maryland Medical Center, 2013)

Mom, be wary of iron. The most common poising emergency in children is accidental iron ingestion. Keep your iron supplements high on a shelf, and in a bullet-proof container. Oh! Why do you have iron supplements around in the first place? If it is for treatment of anemia, that's one thing (and, of course, if this were to be the case, you are taking iron only under medical supervision, right?). If, on the other hand, you are taking iron for some other reason I may have to track you down and get after you.

Treatment for anemia should be directed by your doctor. If you are tired and suspect that you may have anemia, it's important to see your doctor to get a diagnosis, Other conditions can also cause fatigue, and taking iron supplements if you don't need them can be dangerous. (University of Maryland Medical Center, 2013)

Conclusion

Diagnosing maternal thyroid dysfunction during all states of pregnancy is very important for the outcome for both mother and fetus. ~**Feldt-Rasmussen et al., 2011**

With all the fuss over Baby, perhaps I did not pay enough attention to you. You are at risk, too, from the cumulative effects of iodine deficiency and from thyroid hormone issues that arise both before and during pregnancy. For example: _"Up to 20–40% of women with positive thyroid autoantibodies develop hypothyroidism during or immediately after pregnancy...."_ (Männistö, 2013)

As if you need more trouble!—raising a baby, or two, or three, or four, or . . . is challenging enough—no wonder you are so tired all the time! But your tiredness may be due to something else. You may have acquired what is called postpartum thyroid dysfunction (PPTD)—a serious condition that could have been avoided, or at least anticipated, if you had been placed on your physician's radar screen with careful, comprehensive screening for thyroid dysfunction both before or during pregnancy. Beware, there are certain complications that await you . . . at around 13 to 19 weeks postpartum (Lazarus and Premawardhana, 2005). Could it be PPDT?

The early hyperthyroid phase of PPTD causes minimal symptoms and hardly ever requires specific treatment.
However, the hypothyroid phase which occurs later often

needs to be treated with thyroxin [T4] for up to 9 months. A significant number of subjects who have hypothyroid PPTD remain so at the end of the first postpartum year and require long-term thyroxin replacement. (Adlan and Premawardhana, 2011)

I am sharing this with you for a reason. Since PPTD occurs in approximately 1 out of 20 women postpartum, you should probably be screened for this, too. *"Proponents of screening for PPTD justify it on the basis that it is relatively common, causes considerable morbidity, and can be diagnosed with freely available tests that are inexpensive."* (Lazarus and Premawardhana, 2005) Furthermore, of all ladies who make babies, and who, at the same time, make antithyroid antibodies, 50% will develop PPTD after giving birth (Lazarus and Premawardhana, 2005). And if that's not enough bad news for one day, if the postpartum lady's iodine intake is low, as measured by a low urinary excretion of iodine, a higher incidence of PPTD, and perhaps a more aggressive PPTD, can be predicted (Stucky et al., 2011). If you are not feeling well, you are depressed, you are going insane, ask your physician to evaluate you to see if you are experiencing this rather common, serious medical condition.

But enough of this stuff! Now back to Baby, the one who will eventually need piano lessons.

What I have shared with you in the pages of this book is really all about the future. The future *is* universal screening, careful screening for thyroid hormone issues that can harm Baby, destroy Baby, and even harm mothers who want none of this. They have something else in mind. Their heart's desire is the very best start in life for little Jimmy, little Susie, or little whomever—precious little babies who have the right to a healthy start to a happy life. Why not give them every opportunity we can for this to become a reality? Universal screening will help. Why not find <u>all</u> who are at risk? Universal screening, along with timely, appropriate medical intervention, as indicated, will save babies and offer the most vulnerable a chance for the best life has to offer. I've done all I can do here. I've given this book my heart and my soul. Now the rest is up to you.

~Eugene L. Heyden, RN

~Acknowledgments~

I wish to thank the following people who helped make this book possible: First and foremost, my dear wife Toni, who encouraged me along the way while I was writing this little book . . . just for you. I extend a special thanks to Gail Leong and Sandy Keno, both medical librarians at Providence Sacred Heart, Spokane, Washington. I also wish to thank my editor and proofreader, Jacquelyn Barnes.

~References~

Preface

Burman KD 2009 Controversies Surrounding Pregnancy, Maternal Thyroid Status, and Fetal Outcome. Thyroid 19(4):323–326

Delange F 2001 Iodine Deficiency as a Cause of Brain Damage. Postgrad Med J 77:217–220

Dunn JT, Delange F 2001 Damaged Reproduction: The Most Important Consequence of Iodine Deficiency. The Journal of Clinical Investigation 86(6):2360–2363

Moleti M, Presti VPL, Campolo MC, Mattina F, Galletti M, Mandolfino M, Violi MA, et al 2008 Iodine Prophylaxis Using Iodized Salt and Risk of Maternal Thyroid Failure in Conditions of Mild Iodine Deficiency. J Clin Endocrinol Metab; July; 93(7):2616–2621

Nucera C 2010 Maternal Thyroid Hormone Action during Embryo-Fetal Development. Hot Thyroidology (www.hotthyroidology.com) HT 11/1

Introduction

Morreale de Escobar G, Obregón MJ, Escobar del Ray E 2004 Role of Thyroid Hormone during Early Brain Development. European Journal of Endocrinology 151:U25–U37

Neves FA, Cavalieri RR, Simeoni LA, Gardner DG, Baxter JD, Scharschmidt BF, Lomri N, Ribeiro RC 2002 Thyroid Hormone Export Varies Among Primary Cells and Appears to Differ from Hormone Uptake. Endocrinology 143(2):476–483

Obican SG, Jahnke GD, Soldin OP, Scialli AR 2012 Teratology Public Affairs Committee Position Paper: Iodine Deficiency in Pregnancy. Birth Defects Research (Part A) 94:677–682

Paquette MA, Dong H, Gagné R, Williams A, Malowany M, Wade MG, Qauk CL 2011 Thyroid Hormone-Regulated Gene Expression in Juvenile Mouse Liver: Identification of Thyroid Response Elements using Microarray Profiling and *in silico* Analyses. BMC Genomics 12:634

Wang W, Teng W, Shan Z, Wang S, Li J, Zhu L, Zhou J, et al 2011 The Prevalence of Thyroid Disorders during Early Pregnancy in China: The Benefits of Universal Screening in the First Trimester of Pregnancy. European Journal of Endocrinology 164:263–268

Zimmerman M, Delange F 2004 Iodine Supplementation of Pregnant Women in Europe: A Review and Recommendations. European Journal of Clinical Nutrition 58:979–984

Chapter 1 (It's all about you)

Casey BM, Dashe JS, Wells CE, McIntire DD, Byrd W, Leveno KJ, Cunningham FG 2005 Subclinical Hypothyroidism and Pregnancy Outcomes. Obstet Gynecol; February; 105(2):239–245

Feldt-Rasmussen R, Mortensen A-S B, Rasmussen AK, Boas M, Hilsted L, Main K 2011 Challenges in Interpretation of Thyroid Function Tests in Pregnant Women with Autoimmune Thyroid Disease. Journal of Thyroid Research Aritcle ID 598712 doi:10.4061/2011/589712

Hall DR 2009 Abrupto Placentae and Disseminated Intravascular Coagulopathy. Semin Perinatol 33:189–195

Lockwood CJ 2013 Should Pregnant Women Receive Iodine Supplementation? CONTEMPORARYOBGYN.NET; February; 4–6

Morreale de Escobar G, Obregón MJ, Escobar del Ray E 2004 Role of Thyroid Hormone during Early Brain Development. European Journal of Endocrinology 151:U25–U37

Nucera C 2010 Maternal Thyroid Hormone Action during Embryo-Fetal Development. Hot Thyroidology (www.hotthyroidology.com) HT 11/10

Román GC, Ghassabian A, Bingers-Schokking JJ, Jaddoe V, Hofman A, de Rijke YB, Verhuslt FC, Tiemeier H 2013 Association of Gestational Maternal Hypothyroxinemia and Increased Autism Risk. Ann Neurol 74:733–742

Tudosa R, Vartej P, Hornoianu I, Ghica C, Mateescu SM, Dumitrache I 2010 Maternal and Fetal Complications of the Hypothyroidism-Related Pregnancy. Maedica 5(2):116–123

Wang W, Teng W, Shan Z, Wang S, Li J, Zhu L, Zhou J, et al 2011 The Prevalence of Thyroid Disorders during Early Pregnancy in China: The Benefits of Universal Screening in the First Trimester of Pregnancy. European Journal of Endocrinology 164:263–268

Chapter 2 (Just as it should be)

Akinci A, Sarac K, Güngör S, Mungan I, Aydin Ö 2006 Brain MR Spectroscopy Findings in Neonates with Hypothyroidism Born to Mothers Living in Iodine-Deficient Areas. Am J Neuroradiol; Nov–Dec; 27:2083–2087

Allen WC, Haddow JE, Palomaki GE, Williams JR, Mitchell ML, Hermos JR, Faix JD, Klein RZ 2000 Maternal Thyroid Deficiency and Pregnancy Complications: Implications for Population Screening. J Med Screen 7:127–130

Calvo RM, Jauniaux E, Gulbis B, Asunción M, Gervy C, Contempré B, Morreale de Escobar G 2002 Fetal Tissues are Exposed to Biologically Relevant Free Thyroxine Concentrations during Early Phases of Development. The Journal of Clinical Endocrinology & Metabolism 87(4):1768–1777

Dunn JT, Delange F 2001 Damaged Reproduction: The Most Important Consequence of Iodine Deficiency. The Journal of Clinical Investigation 86(6):2360–2363

Ghirri P, Lunardi S, Boldrini A 2014 Iodine Supplementation in the Newborn. Nutrients 6:382–390

Huang SA, Dorfman DM, Genest DR, Salvatore D, Larsen PR 2003 Type 3 Iodothyronne Deiodinase Is Highly Expressed in Human Uroplacental Unit and in Epithelium. The Journal of Clinical Endocrinology & Metabolism 88(3):1384–1388

Kester MHA, Martinez R, de Mena RM, Obregon MJ, Marinkovic D, Howatson A, Visser TJ, Hume R, Morreale de Escobar G 2004 Iodothyronine Levels in the Human Developing Brain: Major

Regulatory Roles of Iodothyronine Deiodinases in Different Areas. The Journal of Clinical Endocrinology & Metabolism 89(7):3117–3128

Mayo Clinic 1998–2014 Hashimoto's Disease. http://www.mayoclinic.org/diseases-conditions/hashimotos-disease/basics/complications/con-20030293

Mitchell ML, Klein RZ 2004 The Sequelae of Untreated Maternal Hypothyroidism. European Journal of Endocrinology 151:U45–U48

Moleti M, Presti VPL, Mattina F, Mancuso A, De Vivo A, Giorgianni G, Di Bella B, et al 2009 Gestational Thyroid Function Abnormalities in Conditions of Mild Iodine Deficiency: Early Screening versus Continuous Monitoring of Maternal Thyroid Status. European Journal of Endocrinology 160:611–617

Nagey DA 2002 Thyroid Disease Raises Risk for Birth Defects. http://www.hopkinsmedicine.org/press/2002/JANUARY/020117.htm

Ozdemir G, Akman I, Coskun S, Demirel U, Turan S, Bereket A, Bilgen H, Ozek E 2013 Maternal Thyroid Dyrfunction and Neonatal Thyroid Problems. International Journal of Endocrinology Article ID 987843

Palha JA, Goodman AB 2005 Thyroid Hormones and Retinoids: A Possible Link between Genes and Environment in Schizophrenia. Brain Research News 51(1):61–71

Román GC, Ghassabian A, Bingers-Schokking JJ, Jaddoe V, Hofman A, de Rijke YB, Verhuslt FC, Tiemeier H 2013 Association of Gestational Maternal Hypothyroxinemia and Increased Autism Risk. Ann Neurol 74:733–742

Stagnaro-Green A, Sullivan S, Pearce EN 2012 Iodine Supplementation during Pregnancy and Lactation. JAMA; December; 308(23):2463–2464

Sutandar M, Garcia-Bournissen F, Koren G 2007 Hypothyroidism in Pregnancy. J Obstet Gynaecol Can; April; 29(4):354–356

Verma I, Sood R, Juneja S, Kaur S 2012 Prevalence of Hypothyroidism in Infertile Women and Evaluation of Response of Treatment for Hypothyroidism on Infertility. Ind J Appl Basic Med Res; January–June; 2(1):17–18

Wasserman EE, Nelson K, Rose NR, Eaton W, Pillion JP, Seaberg E, Taylor MV, et al 2007 Maternal Thyroid Autoantibodies during the

Third Trimester and Hearing Deficits in Children: An Epidemiologic Assessment. Am J Epidemiol 167:701–710

Wikipedia 2014 Amniotic Fluid.
http://en.wikipedia.org/wiki/Amniotic_fluid

Yang H, Shao N, Chen L, Chen Q, Yu L, Cai L, Lin Z, et al 2014 Screening Strategies for Thyroid Disorders in the First Trimester of Pregnancy. PLOS ONE; June; 9(6):e99611

Chapter 3 (What *ever* could go wrong?)

Abraham GE 2003 Iodine Supplementation Markedly Increases Urinary Excretion of Fluoride and Bromide. Townsend Letter 238:108–109. Accessed from:
http://www.wachters.com/printarticle.php?newsID=109

Adlin V 1998 Subclinical Hypothyroidism: Deciding when to treat. Am Fam Physician; February 15; 57(4):776–780

Akinci A, Sarac K, Güngör S, Mungan I, Aydin Ö 2006 Brain MR Spectroscopy Findings in Neonates with Hypothyroidism Born to Mothers Living in Iodine-Deficient Areas. Am J Neuroradiol; Nov–Dec; 27:2083–2087

Alexander EK 2010 Here's to You, Baby! A Step Forward in Support of Universal Screening of Thyroid Function during Pregnancy. J Clin Endrocrinol Metab; April; 95(4):1575–1577

Ausó E Lavado-Autrei R, Cuevas E, Escobar del Rey R, Morreale de Escobar G, Berbel P 2004 A Moderate and Transient Deficiency of Maternal Thyroid Function at the Beginning of Fetal Neocorticogenesis Alters Neuronal Migration. Endocrinology 145(9):4037–4047

Benhadi N, Wiersinga WM, Reitsma JB, Vrijhotte TGM, Bonsel GJ 2009 Higher Maternal TSH Levels in Pregnancy are Associated with Increased Risk for Miscarriage, Fetal or Neonatal Death. European Journal of Endocrinology 160:985–991

Berbel P, Nestre JL, Santamaría AM, Palazón I, Franco A, Graells M, González-Torga A, Morreale de Escobar G 2009 Delayed Neurobehavioral Development in Children Born to Pregnant Women with Mild Hypothyroxinemia during the First Month of Gestation: The Importance of Early Iodine Supplementation. Thyroid 19(5):511–519

Berbel P, Navarro D, Ausó E, Varea E, Rodriguez J, Ballesta JJ, Slainas N, et al 2010 Role of Late Maternal Thyroid Hormones in Cerebral Cortex Development: An Experimental Model for Human Prematurity. Cerebral Cortex; June; 20(6):1462–1475

Bernal J 2014 Thyroid Hormones in Brain Development and Function. Thyroid Disease Manager; Last update December 17, 2012; http://www.thyroidmanager.org/chapter/thyroid-hormones-in-brain-development-and-function/

Casey BM, Dashe JS, Wells CE, McIntire DD, Byrd W, Leveno KJ, Cunningham FG 2005 Subclinical Hypothyroidism and Pregnancy Outcomes. Obstet Gynecol; February; 105(2):239–245

CerebralPalsy.Org 2014 Cost of Cerebral Palsy. http://cerebralplasy.org/about-cerebral-palsy/cost-of-cerebral-palsy/

Cignini P, Cafà EV, Giorlandino C, Caprigliome S, Spata A, Dugo N 2012 Thyroid Physiology and Common Diseases in Pregnancy: Review of Literature. Journal of Prenatal Medicine 6(4):64–71

Diamanti-Kandarakis E, Bourguignon J-P, Giudice LC, Hauser R, Prins GS, Soto AM, Zoeller RT, Gore AC 2009 Endocrine-Disrupting Chemicals: An Endocrine Society Scientific Statement. Endocrine Reviews; June; 30(4):293–342

Dunn JT, Delange F 2001 Damaged Reproduction: The Most Important Consequence of Iodine Deficiency. The Journal of Clinical Investigation 86(6):2360–2363

Feldt-Rasmussen R, Mortensen A-S B, Rasmussen AK, Boas M, Hilsted L, Main K 2011 Challenges in Interpretation of Thyroid Function Tests in Pregnant Women with Autoimmune Thyroid Disease. Journal of Thyroid Research Aritcle ID 598712 doi:10.4061/2011/589712

Ghirri P, Dini F, Boldrini A 2013 Babies Born to Mothers with Thyroid Disease. Early Human Development 89S4:S66–S67

Ghirri P, Lunardi S, Boldrini A 2014 Iodine Supplementation in the Newborn. Nutrients 6:382–390

Glinoer D, Smallridge RC 2004 The Impact of Maternal Thyroid Disease on the Developing Fetus: Implications for Diagnosis, Treatment and Screening. Hot Thyroidology; April; (1):1–6

Glinoer D, Abalovich M 2007 Unresolved Questions in Managing Hypothyroidism during Pregnancy. BMJ; August 11; 355:300–335

Hendrichs J, Bongers-Schokking JJ, Schenk JJ, Ghassabian A, Schmidt HG, Visser, TJ, Hooijkaas H, et al 2010 Maternal Thyroid Function during Early Pregnancy and Cognitive Functioning in Early Childhood: The Generation R Study. J Clin Endocrinol Metab 96:4227–4234

Hendrichs J, Ghassabiant A, Peeters RP, Tiemeiert H 2013 Maternal Hypothyroxinemia and Effects on Cognitive Functioning in Childhood: How and Why? Clinical Endocrinology 79:152–162

Holick MF 2004 Vitamin D: Importance in the Prevention of Cancers, Type 1 Diabetes, Heart Disease, and Osteoporosis. American Journal of Clinical Nutrition; March; 79(3):362–371

Hollowell JG, Hannon WH 1997 Teratogen Update: Iodine Deficiency, a Community Teratogen. Teratology 55:389–405

Kaushal M, Magon N 2013 Vitamin D in Pregnancy: A Metabolic Outlook. Indian J Endocrinol Metab; January–February; 17(1):76–82

Klubo-Gwiezdzinska J, Burman KD, Van Nostrand D, Wartofsky L 2011 Levothyroxin Treatment in Pregnancy: Indications, Efficacy, and Therapeutic Regimen. Journal of Thyroid Research doi:10.4061/2011/843591

Kooistra L, Crawford S, van Baar AL, Brouwers EP, Pop VJ 2006 Neonatal Effects of Maternal Hypothyroxinemia during Early Pregnancy. Pediatrics 117(1):161–167

Leung AM, Pearce EN 2007 Iodine Nutrition in North America. Hot Thyroidology (www.hotthyroidology.com); September; 5

Mandel SJ, Cooper DS 2001 The Use of Antithyroid Drugs in Pregnancy and Lactation. The Journal of Clinical Endocrinology & Metabolism 86(6):2354–2359

Männistö T 2013 Thyroid Disease during Pregnancy. http://www.medscape.com/view article/814179_print

Matuszek B, Zakoscielna Baszak-Radomanska E, Pyzik A, Nowakowski A 2011 Universal Screening as a Recommendation for Thyroid Tests in Pregnant Women. Annals of Agricultural and Environmental Medicine 18(2):375–379

MAYO CLINIC 1998–2014 Pregnancy Week by Week
http://www.mayoclinic.org/healthy-living/pregnancy-week-by-week/in-depth/pregnancy-and-obesity/art-20044409?pg=2&p=1

Moleti M, Presti VPL, Mattina F, Mancuso A, De Vivo A, Giorgianni G, Di Bella B, et al 2009 Gestational Thyroid Function Abnormalities in Conditions of Mild Iodine Deficiency: Early Screening versus Continuous Monitoring of Maternal Thyroid Status. European Journal of Endocrinology 160:611–617

Morreale de Escobar G, Obregón MJ, Escobar del Ray E 2000 Is Neuropsychological Development Related to Maternal Hypothyroidism or to Maternal Hypothyroxinemia? The Journal of Clinical Endocrinology & Metabolism 85(11):3975–3987

Morreale de Escobar G, Obregón MJ, Escobar del Ray E 2004 Role of Thyroid Hormone during Early Brain Development. European Journal of Endocrinology 151:U25–U27

Morreale de Escobar G, Obregón MJ, Escobar del Rey F 2007 Iodine Deficiency and Brain Development in the First Half of Pregnancy. Public Health Nutrition 10(12A):1554–1570

National Institute of Neurological Disorders and Stroke 1996 Study Links Neonatal Thyroid Function to Cerebral Palsy. Press release of Wednesday, March 27

Negro R, Formoso G, Mangieri T, Pezzarossa A, Dazzi D, Hassan H 2006 Levothyronine Treatment in Euthyroid Pregnant Women with Autoimmune Thyroid Disease: Effects on Obstetrical Complications. The Journal of Clinical Endocrinology & Metabolism 91(7):2587–2591

Nelson KB 2009 Preventing Cerebral Palsy: Paths Not (Yet) Taken. Developmental Medicine & Child Neurology 51:765–769

Nucera C 2010 Maternal Thyroid Hormone Action during Embryo-Fetal Development. Hot Thyroidology (www.hotthyroidology.com) HT 11/10

NYTimes.com 2012 F.D.A Makes It Official: BPA Can't Be Used in Baby Bottles and Cups; July 17;
http://www.nytimes.com/2012/07/18/science/fda-bans-bpa-from-baby-bottles-and-sippy-cups.html?_r=2&

Obican SG, Jahnke GD, Soldin OP, Scialli AR 2012 Teratology Public Affairs Committee Position Paper: Iodine Deficiency in Pregnancy. Birth Defects Research (Part A) 94:677–682

Ogilvy-Stuart AL 2002 Neonatal Thyroid Disorders. Arch Dis Child Fetal Neonatal Ed 87:F165–F171

Opazo MC, Gianini A, Pancetti F, Azkcona G, Alarcón L, Lizana R, Noches V, et al 2008 Maternal Hypothyroxinemia Impairs Spatial Learning and Synaptic Nature and Function in the Offspring. Endocrinology 149:5097–5197

Ozdemir G, Akman I, Coskun S, Demirel U, Turan S, Bereket A, Bilgen H, Ozek E 2013 Maternal Thyroid Dysfunction and Neonatal Thyroid Problems. Internaltional Journal of Endocrinology Article ID 987843

Rastogi MV, LaFranchi SH 2010 Congenital Hypothyroidism. Orphanet Journal of Rare Diseases 5(17)

Reuss ML, Paneth N, Pinto-Martin JA, Lornza JM, Susser M 1996 The Relation of Transient Hypothyroxinemia Preterm Infants to Neurologic Development at Two Years of Age. N Engl J Med 334:821–827

Román GC 2007 Autism: Transient *In Utero* Hypothyroxinemia Related to Maternal Flavonoid Ingestion during Pregnancy and to Other Environmental Antithyroid Agents. Journal of Neurological Sciences 262:15–26

Sahay RK, Sir Nagesh VS 2012 Hypothyroidism in Pregnancy. Indian J Endocrinol Metab; May–June; 16(3):364–370

Seror J, Amand G, Guibourdenche J, Ceccaldi P-F, Luton D 2014 Anti-TPO Antibodies Diffusion through the Placental Barrier during Pregnancy. PLOS ONE; January; 9(1):e84647

Skeaff SA 2011 Iodine Deficiency in Pregnancy: The Effect on Neurodevelopment in the Child. Nutrients 3:265–273

Stagnaro-Green A 2011 Thyroid Antibodies and Miscarriage: Where Are We at a Generation Later? Journal of Thyroid Research doi: 10.4061/2011/841949

Thangaratinam S, Tan A, Knox E, Kilby MD, Franklyn J, Coomarasamy A 2011 Association between Thyroid Autoantibodies and Miscarriage and Preterm Birth: Meta-Analysis of Evicence. BMJ 2012;34222:d2616

University of Kansas Medical Center School of Integrative Medicine 2013 Iodine Supplementation. http://www.kumc.edu/school-of-medicine/integrative-medicine/iodine-supplementation.html

Verheesen RH, Schweitzer CM 2008 Iodine Deficiency, More than Cretinism, and Goiter. Medical Hypotheses 71:645–648

Wasserman EE, Nelson K, Rose NR, Eaton W, Pillion JP, Seaberg E, Taylor MV, et al 2007 Maternal Thyroid Autoantibodies during the Third Trimester and Hearing Deficits in Children: An Epidemiologic Assessment. Am J Epidemiol 167:701–710

*Web*MD 2013 Brominated Vegetable Oil Q&A. http://www.webmd.com/food-recipes/news/20130129/brominated-vegetable-oil-qa

Wilson KL, Casey BM, McIntire DD, Halvorson LM, Cunningham FG 2012 Subclinical Thyroid Disease and the Incidence of Hypertension in Pregnancy. Obstetrics & Gynecology; February; 119(2, Part 1):315–320

Yarrington C, Pearce EN 2011 Iodine and Pregnancy. Journal of Thyroid Research doi:10.4061/2011/934104

Yassa L, Marqusee E, Fawcett R, Alexander EK 2010 Thyroid Hormone Early Adjustment in Pregnancy (The THERAPY) Trial. J Clin Endocrinol Metab 95:3234–3241

Yu X, Chen Y, Shan Z, Teng W, Li C, Zhou W, Gao B, et al 2013 The Pattern of Thyroid Function of Subclinical Hypothyroid Women with Levothyroxine Treatment during Pregnancy. Endocrine 44:710–715

Zimmermann N, Delange R 2004 Iodine Supplementation of Pregnant Women in Europe: A Review and Recommendations. European Journal of Clinical Nutrition 58:979–984

Zoeller RT, Rovet J 2004 Timing of Thyroid Hormone Action in the Developing Brain: Clinical Observations and Experiential Findings. Journal of Neuroendocrinology 16:809–818

Chapter 4 (The impact of iodine deficiency)

Berbel P, Mestre JL, Santamaría A, Palazón I, Franco A, Graells M, González-Torga A, de Escobar GM 2009 Delayed Neurobehavioral Development in Children Born to Pregnant Women with Mild

Hypothyroxinemia during the First Month of Gestation: The Importance of Early Iodine Supplementation. Thyroid, May; 19(5):511–519

Delange F 2001 Iodine Deficiency as a Cause of Brain Damage. Postgrad Med J 77:217–220

Dunn JT, Delange F 2001 Damaged Reproduction: The Most Important Consequence of Iodine Deficiency. The Journal of Clinical Investigation 86(6):2360–2363

Gronowski AM 2012 Thyroid Function during Pregnancy: Who and How We Screen? Clinical Chemistry 58:10
doi/10.1373/clinchem.2012.185017

Hollowell JG, Hannon WH 1997 Teratogen Update: Iodine Deficiency, a Community Teratogen. Teratology 55:389–405

Hong T, Paneth N 2008 Maternal and Infant Thyroid Disorders and Cerebral Palsy. Semin Perinatol 32:438–445

Matuszek B, Zakoscielna Baszak-Radomanska E, Pyzik A, Nowakowski A 2011 Universal Screening as a Recommendation for Thyroid Tests in Pregnant Women. Annals of Agricultural and Environmental Medicine 18(2):375–379

Morreale de Escobar G, Obregón MJ, Escobar del Rey F 2007 Iodine Deficiency and Brain Development in the First Half of Pregnancy. Public Health Nutrition 10(12A):1554–1570

Negro R, Soldin OP, Obregon M-J, Stagnaro-Green A 2011 Hypothyroxinemia and Pregnancy. Endocrine Practice; May/June; 17(3):422–429

Román GC 2007 Autism: Transient *In Utero* Hypothyroxinemia Related to Maternal Flavonoid Ingestion during Pregnancy and to Other Environmental Antithyroid Agents. Journal of Neurological Sciences 262:15–26

Sarici D, Ali M, Kurtoglu S, Akin L, Tucer B, Yikilmaz A, Gokoglu A 2013 Iodine Deficiency: A Probable Cause of Neural Tube Defects. Childs Nerv Syst 29:1027–1030

Skeaff SA 2011 Iodine Deficiency in Pregnancy: The Effect on Neurodevelopment in the Child. Nutrients 3:265–273

Verheesen RH, Schweitzer CM 2008 Iodine Deficiency, More than Cretinism, and Goiter. Medical Hypotheses 71:645–648

Chapter 5 (The myth of iodine sufficiency)

Bo S, Menato G, Villois P; Gambino R, Cassader M, Cotrino I, Cavallo-Perin P 2009 Iron Supplementation and Gestational Diabetes in Midpregnancy. American Journal of Obstetrics & Gynecology, August; 201:158.e1–6

Charles D HM, Ness AR, Campbell D, Smith GD, Whitley E, Hall MH 2005 Folic Acid Supplementation in Pregnancy and Birth Outcome: Re-Analysis of a Large Randomized Controlled Trial and Update of Cochrane Review. Paediatric and Perinatal Epidemiology 19:112–124

Delange F 2004 Optimal Iodine Nutrition during Pregnancy, Lactation and the Neonatal Period. Int J Endocrinol Metab 2:1–12

Dunn JT, Delange F 2001 Damaged Reproduction: The Most Important Consequence of Iodine Deficiency. The Journal of Clinical Investigation 86(6):2360–2363

Helin A, Kinnunen TI, Raitanen J, Ahonen S, Virtanen SM, Luoto R 2012 Iron Intake, Haemoglobin and Risk of Gestational Diabetes: A Prospective Cohort Study. BMJ Open2:e0017730

Hollowell JG, Hannon WH 1997 Teratogen Update: Iodine Deficiency, a Community Teratogen. Teratology 55:389–405

Hollowell JG, Haddow JE 2007 The Prevalence of Iodine Deficiency in Women of Reproductive Age in the United States of America. Public Health Nutrition 10(12A):1532–1539

Hwang J-Y, Lee J-Y, Kim K-N, Kim H, Ha E-H, Park H, Ha M, et al 2013 Maternal Iron Intake at Mid-Pregnancy Is Associated with Reduced Fetal Growth: Results from Mothers and Children's Environmental Health (MOCEH) Study. Nutritional Journal 12:38

Leung AM, Pearce EN 2007 Iodine Nutrition in North America. Hot Thyroidology (www.hotthyroidology.com); September; 5

Leung AM, LaMar A, He X, Braverman LE, Pearce EN 2011 Iodine Status and Thyroid Function of Boston-Area Vegetarians and Vegans. J Clin Endocrinol Metab; August; 96(8):E1303–1307

Lockwood CJ 2013 Should Pregnant Women Receive Iodine Supplementation? CONTEMPORARYOBGYN.NET; February 2; 4–6

Morreale de Escobar G, Obregón MJ, Escobar del Ray E 2004 Role of Thyroid Hormone during Early Brain Development. European Journal of Endocrinology 151:U25–U27

Pearce EN, Pino S, He X, Bazrafshan HR, Lee SL, Braverman LE 2004 Sources of Dietary Iodine: Bread, Cows' Milk, and Infant Formula in the Boston Area. The Journal of Clinical Endocrinology & Metabolism 89(7):3421–3424

Scholl TO 2005 Iron Status during Pregnancy: Setting the Stage for Mother and Infant. Am J Clin Nutr 81(suppl):1218S–1222S

Skeaff SA 2011 Iodine Deficiency in Pregnancy: The Effect on Neurodevelopment in the Child. Nutrients 3:265–273

Smyth PPA, Duntas LH 2005 Iodine Uptake and Loss—Can Frequent Strenuous Exercise Induce Iodine Deficiency? Horm Metab Res 37:555–558

Stagnaro-Green A, Pearce E 2012 Thyroid Disorders in Pregnancy. Nat. Rev. Endocrinol 8:650–658

Thompson MD, Cole D EC, Ray JG 2009 Vitamin B-12 and Neural Tube Defects: The Canadian Experience. Am J Clin Nutr 89(suppl):697–701

Verheesen RH, Schweitzer CM 2008 Iodine Deficiency, More than Cretinism and Goiter. Med Hypothesis; November; 71(5):645–648

*Web*MD, 2009 Birth Defects Linked to Low Vitamin B12. http://www.webmd.com/baby/news/20090302/birth-defects-linked-to-low-vitamin-b12

Yarrington C, Pearce EN 2011 Iodine and Pregnancy. Journal of Thyroid Research doi:10.4061/2011/934104

Ziaei S, Norrozi M, Faghihzadeh S, Jafarbegloo E 2007 A Randomized Placebo-Controlled Trial to Determine the Effect of Iron Supplementation on Pregnancy Outcomes in Pregnant Women with Haemoglobin $\geq$ 13.2 g/dl. BLOG 114:684–688

Chapter 6 (You will be missed)

Akinci A, Sarac K, Güngör S, Mungan I, Aydin Ö 2006 Brain MR Spectroscopy Findings in Neonates with Hypothyroidism Born to Mothers Living in Iodine-Deficient Areas. Am J Neuroradiol; Nov–Dec; 27:2083–2087

Alexander EK 2010 Here's to You, Baby! A Step Forward in Support of Universal Screening of Thyroid Function during Pregnancy. J Clin Endrocrinol Metab; April; 95(4):1575–1577

Allan WC, Haddow JE, Palomaki GE, Williams JR, Mitchell ML, Hermos JR, Faix JD, Klein RZ 2000 Maternal Thyroid Deficiency and Pregnancy Complications: Implications for Population Screening. J Med Screen 7:127–130

American Association of Clinical Chemistry 2012 Thyroid Function during Pregnancy: Who and How Should We Screen? (Podcast) http://www.aacc.org/publications/clin_chem/podcast/Documents/Cli nChem201210_Gronowski-Haddow.pdf

American Thyroid Association 2013 The Case for Universal Screening in Pregnancy. http://www.thyroid.org/the-case-for-universal-thyroid-screening-in-pregnancy/

Bernal J 2014 Thyroid Hormones in Brain Development and Function. Thyroid Disease Manager; Last update December 17, 2012; http://www.thyroidmanager.org/chapter/thyroid-hormones-in-brain-development-and-function/

Brent GA 2007 Diagnosing Thyroid Dysfunction in Pregnant Women: Is Case Finding Enough? The Journal of Clinical Endocrinology & Metabolism 92(1):39–41

Dosiou C, Sanders G, Araki SS, Crapo LM 2008 Screening Pregnant Women for Autoimmune Thyroid Disease: A Cost-Effective Analysis. European Journal of Endocrinology 158:841–851

Feldt-Rasmussen R, Mortensen A-S B, Rasmussen AK, Boas M, Hilsted L, Main K 2011 Challenges in Interpretation of Thyroid Function Tests in Pregnant Women with Autoimmune Thyroid Disease. Journal of Thyroid Research Article ID 598712 doi:10.4061/2011/589712

Gronowski AM 2012 Thyroid Function during Pregnancy: Who and How We Screen? Clinical Chemistry 58:10 doi:10.1373/clinchem.2012.185017

Hendrichs J, Bongers-Schokking JJ, Schenk JJ, Ghassabian A, Schmidt HG, Visser, TJ, Hooijkaas H, et al 2010 Maternal Thyroid Function during Early Pregnancy and Cognitive Functioning in Early Childhood: The Generation R Study. J Clin Endocrinol Metab 96:4227–4234

Jiskra J, BartáKová J, Holomka Š, Límanová Z, Springer D, Antošová M, Telička Z, Potluková E 2011 Low Prevalence of Clinically High-Risk Women and Pathological Thyroid Ultrasound among Pregnant Women Positive in Universal Screening for Thyroid Disorders. Experimental and Clinical Endocrinology and Diabetes 119(9):530

Lepoutre T, Debiève F, Gruson D, Daumerie C 2012 Reduction of Miscarriages through Universal Screening and Treatment of Thyroid Autoimmune Diseases. Gynecol Obstet Invest 74:365–273

Matuszek B, Zakoscielna Baszak-Radomanska E, Pyzik A, Nowakowski A 2011 Universal Screening as a Recommendation for Thyroid Tests in Pregnant Women. Annals of Agricultural and Environmental Medicine 18(2):375–379

Mitchell ML, Klein RZ 2004 The Sequelae of Untreated Maternal Hypothyroidism. European Journal of Endocrinology 151:U45–U48

Moleti M, Presti VPL, Mattina F, Mancuso A, De Vivo A, Giorgianni G, Di Bella B, et al 2009 Gestational Thyroid Function Abnormalities in Conditions of Mild Iodine Deficiency: Early Screening versus Continuous Monitoring of Maternal Thyroid Status. European Journal of Endocrinology 160:611–617

Negro R, Formoso G, Mangieri T, Pezzarossa A, Dazzi D, Hassan H 2006 Levothyronine Treatment in Euthyroid Pregnant Women with Autoimmune Thyroid Disease: Effects on Obstetrical Complications. The Journal of Clinical Endocrinology & Metabolism 91(7):2587–2591

Nucera C 2010 Maternal Thyroid Hormone Action during Embryo-Fetal Development. Hot Thyroidology (www.hotthyroidology.com) HT 11/10

Opazo MC, Gianini A, Pancetti F, Azkcona G, Alarcón L, Lizana R, Noches V, et al 2008 Maternal Hypothyroxinemia Impairs Spatial

Learning and Synaptic Nature and Function in the Offspring. Endocrinology 149:5097–5197

Sreedharan S, Poulose PK, Kesavan L, Indumathi K 2012 Transplacental Transfer of Antithyroid Antibodies a Preliminary Report. Thyroid Research and Practice; January–April 9(1):7–8

Soldin OP, Chung SH, Colie C 2013 The Use of TSH Determining Thyroid Disease: How Does It Impact the Practice of Medicine in Pregnancy? Journal of Thyroid Research Article ID 148157

Su P-Y, Huang K, Hao J-H, Xu Y-Q, Yam S-Q, Li T, Xu Y-H, Tao F-B 2011 Maternal Thyroid Function in the First Twenty Weeks of Pregnancy and Subsequent Fetal and Infant Development: A Prospective Population-Based Cohort Study in China. J Clin Emndocrinol Metab 96:3234–3241

Vila L, Velasco I, Gonález S, Morales F, Sánchez E, Torrejón S, Soldevial B, et al 2014 On the Need for Universal Thyroid Screening in Pregnant Women. European Journal of Endocrinology 170(1):R17–R30

Wang W, Teng W, Shan Z, Wang S, Li J, Zhu L, Zhou J, et al 2011 The Prevalence of Thyroid Disorders during Early Pregnancy in China: The Benefits of Universal Screening in the First Trimester of Pregnancy. European Journal of Endocrinology 164:263–268

Wasserman EE, Nelson K, Rose NR, Eaton W, Pillion JP, Seaberg E, Taylor MV, et al 2007 Maternal Thyroid Autoantibodies during the Third Trimester and Hearing Deficits in Children: An Epidemiologic Assessment. Am J Epidemiol 167:701–710

Chapter 7 (Spare the children)

Akinci A, Sarac K, Güngör S, Mungan I, Aydin Ö 2006 Brain MR Spectroscopy Findings in Neonates with Hypothyroidism Born to Mothers Lining in Iodine-Deficient Areas. Am J Neuroradiol; Nov–Dec; 27:2083–2087

Alvarez N 2014 Cerebral Palsy. *Web*MD/emedicine*health* http://www.emedicinehealth.com/script/main/art.asp?articlekey=590 56&pf=3&page=1

Ares S, Escobar-Morreale HF, Quero J, Durán S, Presas MJ, Hurruzo J, Morreale de Escobar G 1997 Neonatal Hypothyroxinemia: Effects of

Iodine Intake and Premature Birth. The Journal of Clinical Endocrinology & Metabolism 82(6)1704–1712

Berbel P, Navarro D, Ausó E, Varea E, Rodriguez J, Ballesta JJ, Slainas N, et al 2010 Role of Late Maternal Thyroid Hormones in Cerebral Cortex Development: An Experimental Model for Human Prematurity. Cerebral Cortex; June; 20(6):1462–1475

Bernal J 2014 Thyroid Hormones in Brain Development and Function. Thyroid Disease Manager; Last update December 17, 2012; http://www.thyroidmanager.org/chapter/thyroid-hormones-in-brain-development-and-function/

Boas M, Feldt-Rasmussen U, Main KM 2012 Thyroid Effects of Endocrine Disrupting Chemicals. Molecular and Cellular Endocrinology 355:240–248

Bouhouch RR, Bouhouch S, Cherkaoui M, Aboussad A, Stinca S, Haldimann N, Anderson M, Zimmermann MB 2013 Direct Iodine Supplementation of Infants Versus Supplementation of Their Breastfeeding Mothers: A Double-Blind, Randomized, Placebo-Controlled Trial. The Lancet Diabetes & Endocrinology 2(3):197–209

Calvo RM, Jauniaux E, Gulbis B, Asunción M, Gervy C, Contempré B, Morreale de Escobar G 2002 Fetal Tissues are Exposed to Biologically Relevant Free Thyroxine Concentrations during Early Phases of Development. The Journal of Clinical Endocrinology & Metabolism 87(4):1768–1777

CerebralPalsy.Org 2014 Cost of Cerebral Palsy. http://cerebralpalsy.org/about-cerebral-palsy/cost-of-cerebral-palsy/

Dosiou C, Sanders G, Araki SS, Crapo LM 2008 Screening Pregnant Women for Autoimmune Thyroid Disease: A Cost-Effective Analysis. European Journal of Endocrinology 158:841–851

Haymart MR 2010 The Role of Clinical Guidelines in Patient Care: Thyroid Hormone Replacement in Women of Reproductive Age. Thyroid 20:301–307

Hendrichs J, Bongers-Schokking JJ, Schenk JJ, Ghassabian A, Schmidt HG, Visser, TJ, Hooijkaas H, et al 2010 Maternal Thyroid Function during Early Pregnancy and Cognitive Functioning in Early Childhood: The Generation R Study. J Clin Endocrinol Metab 96:4227–4234

Hendricks J, Ghassabiant A, Peeters RP, Tiemeiert H 2013 Maternal Hypothyroxinemia and Effects on Cognitive Functioning in Childhood: How and Why? Clinical Endocrinology 79:152–162

Hollis BW, Wagner CL 2004 Assessment of Dietary Vitamin D Requirements during Pregnancy and Lactation. Am J Clin Nutr 79:717–726

Hollowell JG, Hannon WH 1997 Teratogen Update: Iodine Deficiency, a Community Teratogen. Teratology 55:389–405

Hollowell JG, Staehling NW, Hannon WH, Flanders DW, Gunter EW, Maberly GF, Braverman LE, et al 1998 Iodine Nutrition in the United States. Trends and Public Health Implications: Iodine Excretion Data from National Health and Nutrition Examination Surveys I and III (1971–1974 and 1988–1994). Journal of Clinical Endocrinology and Metabolism 83(10):3401–3408

John's Hopkins Medicine 2002 Thyroid Disease Raises Risk for Birth Defects
http://www.hopkinsmedicine.org/press/2002/JANUARY/020117.htm

Lemacjs J, Fowles K, Mateus A, Thomas K 2013 Insights from Parents about Caring for a Child with Birth Defects. Int. J. Environ. Res, Public Health 10:3465–3482

Leung AM, Pearce EN, Braverman LE 2011 Iodine Nutrition in Pregnancy and Lactation. Endocrinol Metab Clin North Am; December; 40(4):765–777

Lopez MM 2012 Hypothyroxinemia in Pregnancy is Related with Attention Deficit Hyperactivity Disorder. Contemporary Trends in ASHD Research; Chapter 5; Dr. Jill M Norvilitis (Ed.), ISBN: 978-953-307-858-8

Maberly GF, Haxton DP, van der Haar F 2003 Iodine Deficiency: Consequences and Progress toward Elimination. Food and Nutrition Bulletin 24(4):S91–S98

Männistö T 2013 Thyroid Disease during Pregnancy.
http://www.medscape.com/view article/814179_print

Massachusetts General Hospital 2010 Attention Deficit/Hyperactivity disorder (ADHD).
http://www2.massgeneral.org/schoolpsychiatry/info_adhd.asp

Mayo Clinic 1998–2014 Hashimoto's Disease. http://www.mayoclinic.org/diseases-conditions/hashimotos-disease/basics/complications/con-20030293

Mitchell ML, Klein RZ 2004 The Sequelae of Untreated Maternal Hypothyroidism. European Journal of Endocrinology 151:U45–U48

Moleti M, Presti VPL, Campolo MC, Mattina F, Galletti M, Mandolfino M, Violi MA, et al 2008 Iodine Prophylaxis Using Iodized Salt and Risk of Maternal Thyroid Failure in Conditions of Mild Iodine Deficiency. J Clin Endocrinol Metab; July; 93(7):2616–2621

Morreale de Escobar G, Obregón MJ, Escobar del Ray E 2004 Role of Thyroid Hormone during Early Brain Development. European Journal of Endocrinology 151:U25–U27

Morreale de Escobar G, Obregón MJ, Escobar del Rey F 2007 Iodine Deficiency and Brain Development in the First Half of Pregnancy. Public Health Nutrition 10(12A):1554–1570

National Institute of Neurological Disorders and Stroke 1996 Study Links Neonatal Thyroid Function to Cerebral Palsy. Press release of Wednesday, March 27

Negro R, Formoso G, Mangieri T, Pezzarossa A, Dazzi D, Hassan H 2006 Levothyronine Treatment in Euthyroid Pregnant Women with Autoimmune Thyroid Disease: Effects on Obstetrical Complications. The Journal of Clinical Endocrinology & Metabolism 91(7):2587–2591

Nelson KB 2009 Preventing Cerebral Palsy: Paths Not (Yet) Taken. Developmental Medicine & Child Neurology 51:765–769

Palha JA, Goodman AB 2005 Thyroid Hormones and Retinoids: A Possible Link between Genes and Environment in Schizophrenia. Brain Research News 51(1):61–71

Reuss ML, Paneth N, Pinto-Martin JA, Lornza JM, Susser M 1996 The Relation of Transient Hypothyroxinemia Preterm Infants to Neurologic Development at Two Years of Age. N Engl J Med 334:821–827

Román GC 2007 Autism: Transient *In Utero* Hypothyroxinemia Related to Maternal Flavonoid Ingestion during Pregnancy and to Other Environmental Antithyroid Agents. Journal of Neurological Sciences 262:15–26

Román GC, Ghassabian A, Bingers-Schokking JJ, Jaddoe V, Hofman A, de Rijke YB, Verhuslt FC, Tiemeier H 2013 Association of Gestational Maternal Hypothyroxinemia and Increased Autism Risk. Ann Neurol 74:733–742

Sarici D, Ali M, Kurtoglu S, Akin L, Tucer B, Yikilmaz A, Gokoglu A 2013 Iodine Deficiency: A Probable Cause of Neural Tube Defects. Childs Nerv Syst 29:1027–1030

Shin DY, Kim KJ, Kim D, Hwang S, Lee EJ 2014 Low Serum Vitamin D is Associated with Anti-Thyroid Peroxidase Antibody in Autoimmune Thyroiditis. Yonsei Med J 55(2):476–481

Skeaff SA 2011 Iodine Deficiency in Pregnancy: The Effect on Neurodevelopment in the Child. Nutrients 3:265–273

Su P-Y, Huang K, Hao J-H, Xu Y-Q, Yam S-Q, Li T, Xu Y-H, Tao F-B 2011 Maternal Thyroid Function in the First Twenty Weeks of Pregnancy and Subsequent Fetal and Infant Development: A Prospective Population-Based Cohort Study in China. J Clin Emndocrinol Metab 96:3234–3241

Vermiglio F, Lo Presti VP, Moleti M, Sidoti M, Tortorella G, Scaffidi G, Castagna MG, et al 2004 Attention Deficit and Hyperactivity Disorders in the Offspring of Mothers Exposed to Mild-Moderate Iodine Deficiency: A Possible Novel Iodine Deficiency Disorder in Developed Countries. The Journal of Clinical Endocrinology & Metabolism 89(12):6054–6060

Wang W, Teng W, Shan Z, Wang S, Li J, Zhu L, Zhou J, et al 2011 The Prevalence of Thyroid Disorders during Early Pregnancy in China: The Benefits of Universal Screening in the First Trimester of Pregnancy. European Journal of Endocrinology 164:263–268

Yoon BH, Park C-W, Chaiworapongsa T 2003 Intrauterine Infection and the Development of Cerebral Palsy. BJOG: an International Journal of Obstetrics and Gynaecology; April; 110(suppl 20):124–127

Zoeller RT, Rovet J 2004 Timing of Thyroid Hormone Action in the Developing Brain: Clinical Observations and Experiential Findings. Journal of Neuroendocrinology 16:809–818

Chapter 8 (Recommendations)

Alexander EK 2010 Here's to You, Baby! A Step Forward in Support of Universal Screening of Thyroid Function during Pregnancy. J Clin Endrocrinol Metab; April; 95(4):1575–1577

American Association of Clinical Chemistry 2012 Thyroid Function during Pregnancy: Who and How Should We Screen? (Podcast) http://www.aacc.org/publications/clin_chem/podcast/Documents/ClinChem201210_Gronowski-Haddow.pdf

Delange F 2004 Optimal Iodine Nutrition during Pregnancy, Lactation and the Neonatal Period. Int J Endocrinol Metab 2:1–12

Dunn JT, Delange F 2001 Damaged Reproduction: The Most Important Consequence of Iodine Deficiency. The Journal of Clinical Investigation 86(6):2360–2363

Ghirri P, Dini F, Boldrini A 2013 Babies Born to Mothers with Thyroid Disease. Early Human Development 89S4:S66–S67

Glinoer D, Abalovich M 2007 Unresolved Questions in Managing Hypothyroidism during Pregnancy. BMJ 335:300–302

Glinoer D, Smallridge RC 2004 The Impact of Maternal Thyroid Disease on the Developing Fetus: Implications for Diagnosis, Treatment and Screening. Hot Thyroidology; April; (1):1–6

Gronowski AM 2012 Thyroid Function during Pregnancy: Who and How We Screen? Clinical Chemistry 58:10 doi/10.1373/clinchem.2012.185017

Khandelwal M 2007 What You Need to Know about Thyroid Disorders in Pregnancy OBG Management; May; 27–31 www.obgmanagement.com

Klubo-Gwiezdzinska J, Burman KD, Van Nostrand D, Wartofsky L 2011 Levothyroxin Treatment in Pregnancy: Indications, Efficacy, and Therapeutic Regimen. Journal of Thyroid Research doi:10.4061/2011/843591

Leung AM, Pearce EN 2007 Iodine Nutrition in North America. Hot Thyroidology (www.hotthyroidology.com); September; 5

Leung AM, Pearce EN, Braverman LE 2011 Iodine Nutrition in Pregnancy and Lactation. Endocrinol Metab Clin North Am; December; 40(4):765–777

Männistö T 2013 Thyroid Disease during Pregnancy. http://www.medscape.com/view article/814179_print

March of Dimes 2009 Vitamins and Minerals during Pregnancy. http://www.marchofdimes.com/pregnancy/vitamins-and-minerals-during-pregnancy.aspx

Morreale de Escobar G, Obregón MJ, Escobar del Ray E 2004 Role of Thyroid Hormone during Early Brain Development. European Journal of Endocrinology 151:U25–U27

Morreale de Escobar G, Obregón MJ, Escobar del Rey F 2007 Iodine Deficiency and Brain Development in the First Half of Pregnancy. Public Health Nutrition 10(12A):1554–1570

Ogilvy-Stuart AL 2002 Neonatal Thyroid Disorders. Arch Dis Child Fetal Neonatal Ed 87:F165–F171

Ozdemir G, Akman I, Coskun S, Demirel U, Turan S, Bereket A, Bilgen H, Ozek E 2013 Maternal Thyroid Dysfunction and Neonatal Thyroid Problems. International Journal of Endocrinology Article ID 987843

Pearce EN, Anderson M, Zimmerman MB 2013 Global Iodine Nutrition: Where Do We Stand in 2013? Thyroid 23(5):523–528

Skeaff SA 2011 Iodine Deficiency in Pregnancy: The Effect on Neurodevelopment in the Child. Nutrients 3:265–273

Soldin OP, Chung SH, Colie C 2013 The Use of TSH Determining Thyroid Disease: How Does It Impact the Practice of Medicine in Pregnancy? Journal of Thyroid Research Article ID 148157

Stagnaro-Green A, Abalovich M, Alexander E, Azizi F, Mestman J, Negro R, Nixon A, et al 2011 Guidelines of the American Thyroid Association for the Diagnosis and Management of Thyroid Disease during Pregnancy and Postpartum. Thyroid 21(10):1081–1125

Stagnaro-Green A, Pearce E 2012 Thyroid Disorders in Pregnancy. Nat. Rev. Endocrinol 8:650–658

Teng X, Shan Z, Chen Y, Lai Y, Yu J, Shan L, Bai X, et al 2011 More Than Adequate Iodine Intake May Increase Subclinical Hypothyroidism and Autoimmune Thyroiditis: A Cross-Sectional Study Based on Two

Chinese Communities with Different Iodine Intake Levels. European Journal of Endocrinology 164:943–950

Vandedpas JB, Contempré B, Duale NL, Deckx H, Bebe N, Lonombé AO, Thilly C-H, et al 1993 Selenium Deficiency Mitigates Hypothyroxinemia in Iodine-Deficient Subjects. Am J Nutr Suppl 57(27):1S–5S

Vila L, Velasco I, Gonález S, Morales F, Sánchez E, Torrejón S, Soldevial B, et al 2014 On the Need for Universal Thyroid Screening in Pregnant Women. European Journal of Endocrinology 170(1):R17–R30

Wang W, Teng W, Shan Z, Wang S, Li J, Zhu L, Zhou J, et al 2011 The Prevalence of Thyroid Disorders during Early Pregnancy in China: The Benefits of Universal Screening in the First Trimester of Pregnancy. European Journal of Endocrinology 164:263–268

Wilson KL, Casey BM, McIntire DD, Halvorson LM, Cunningham FG 2012 Subclinical Thyroid Disease and the Incidence of Hypertension in Pregnancy. Obstetrics & Gynecology; February; 119(2, Part 1):315–320

Yarrington C, Pearce EN 2011 Iodine and Pregnancy. Journal of Thyroid Research doi:10.4061/2011/934104

Yassa L, Marqusee E, Fawcett R, Alexander EK 2010 Thyroid Hormone Early Adjustment in Pregnancy (The THERAPY) Trial. J Clin Endocrinol Metab 95:3234–3241

Yu X, Chen Y, Shan Z, Teng W, Li C, Zhou W, Gao B, et al 2013 The Pattern of Thyroid Function of Subclinical Hypothyroid Women with Levothyroxine Treatment during Pregnancy. Endocrine 44:710–715

Ziaei S, Norrozi M, Faghihzadeh S, Jafarbegloo E 2007 A Randomized Placebo-Controlled Trial to Determine the Effect of Iron Supplementation on Pregnancy Outcomes in Pregnant Women with Haemoglobin $\geq$ 13.2 g/dl. BLOG 114:684–688

Zimmerman M, Delange F 2004 Iodine Supplementation of Pregnant Women in Europe: A Review and Recommendations. European Journal of Clinical Nutrition 58:979–984

Zoeller RT, Rovet J 2004 Timing of Thyroid Hormone Action in the Developing Brain: Clinical Observations and Experiential Findings. Journal of Neuroendocrinology 16:809–818

Chapter 9 (New and what to do)

Belfort MB, Pearce EN, Braverman LE, He X, Brown RS 2012 Low Iodine Content in the Diets of Hospitalized Preterm Infants. J Clin Endocrinol Metab 97(4):E632–E636

Berbel P, Navarro D, Ausó E, Varea E, Rodriguez J, Ballesta JJ, Slainas N, et al 2010 Role of Late Maternal Thyroid Hormones in Cerebral Cortex Development: An Experimental Model for Human Prematurity. CerebralCortex; June; 20(6):1462–1475

Biswas S, Buffery J, Enoch H, Bland M, Markiewicz M, Walters D 2003 Pulmonary Effects of Triiodothyronine (T3) and Hydrocortisone (HC) Supplementation in Pereterm Infants less than 30 Weeks Gestation: Results of The THORN Trial—Thyroid Hormone Relplacement in Neonates. Pediatr Res 53(1):48–56

Cools F, van Wassenaer AG, Kok JH, de Vijlder J J M 2000 Changes in Plasma Thyroid Hormone Levels after a Single Dose of Triiodothyrone in Premature Infants of Less than 30 Weeks Gestational Age. European Journal of Endocrinology 143:733–740

Crawford BA, Cowell CT, Emder PJ, Learoyd DL, Chua EL, Sinn J, Jack MM 2010 Iodine Toxicity from Soy Milk and Seaweed Ingestion is Associated with Serious Thyroid Dysfunction. MJA 193:413–415

Feingold SB, Brown RS 2010 Neonatal Thyroid Function. NeoReviews 11(11):e640–e646

Ghirri P, Lunardi S, Boldrini A 2014 Iodine Supplementation in the Newborn. Nutrients 6:382–390

Golombek SG, LaGamma EF, Paneth N 2002 Treatment of Transient Hypothyroxinemia of Prematurity: A Survey of Neonatal Practice. Journal of Perinatology 22:563–565

Ibrahim N, Morreale de Escobar G, Visser TJ, Durán S, van Toor H, Strachan J 2003 Iodine Deficiency Associated with Parenteral Nutrition in Extreme Preterm Infant. Arch Dis Child Fetal Neonatal Ed 88:F56–F57

La Gamma EF, van Wassenaer AG, Ares S, Colombek SG, Kok JH, Quero J, Hiong T et al 2009 Phase 1 Trial or 4 Thyroid Hormone Regimens for Transient Hypothyroxinemia in Neonates of <28 Weeks' Gestation. Pedaitrics; August; 124(2): e258–e268

Leung AM, Pearce EN, Braverman LE 2011 Iodine Nutrition in Pregnancy and Lactation. Endocrinol Metab Clin North Am; December; 40(4):765–777

Männistö T 2013 Thyroid Disease during Pregnancy. http://www.medscape.com/view article/814179_print

McElduff A, McElduff P, Wily V, Wicken B 2005 Neonatal Thyrotropin as Measured in a Congenital Hypothyroidism Screening Program: Influence of the Mode of Delivery. The Journal of Clinical Endocrinology & Metabolism 90(12):6361–6363

Ng SN, Turner MA, Gamble C, Didi A, Victor S, Weidling AM 2008 TIPIT: A Randomised Controlled Trial of Thyroxine in Preterm Infants under 28 Weeks' Gestation. Trial 9:7 doi:10.1186/1745-6215-9-17

Simpser T, Rapaport R 2010 Update on Some Aspects of Neonatal Thyroid Disease. J Clin Ped Endo 2(3):95–99

Ozdemir G, Akman I, Coskun S, Demirel U, Turan S, Bereket A, Bilgen H, Ozek E 2013 Maternal Thyroid Dysfunction and Neonatal Thyroid Problems. International Journal of Endocrinology Article ID 987843

University of Maryland Medical Center 2013 Iron. https://umm.edu/health/medical/altmed/supplement/iron

Zimmermann MB 2009 Iodine Deficiency. Endocrine Reviews; June; 30(4):376–408

Zoeller RT, Rovet J 2004 Timing of Thyroid Hormone Action in the Developing Brain: Clinical Observations and Experiential Findings. Journal of Neuroendocrinology 16:809–818

Conclusion

Adlan MA, Premawardhana LD 2011 Thyroid Peroxidase Antibody and Screening for Postpartum Thyroid Dysfunction. Journal of Thyroid Research doi: 4061/2011/745135

Feldt-Rasmussen R, Mortensen A-S B, Rasmussen AK, Boas M, Hilsted L, Main K 2011 Challenges in Interpretation of Thyroid Function Tests in Pregnant Women with Autoimmune Thyroid Disease. Journal of Thyroid Research Article ID 598712 doi:10.4061/2011/589712

Lazarus JH, Premawardhana LD 2005 Screening for Thyroid Disease in Pregnancy. J Clin Pathol 58:449–452

Männistö T 2013 Thyroid Disease during Pregnancy. http://www.medscape.com/view article/814179_print

Stuckey BGA, Kent GN, Allen RJ, Ward LC, Brown SJ, Walsh JP 2011 Low Urinary Iodine Postpartum is Associated with Hypothyroid Postpartum Thyroid Dysfunction and Predicts Long-term Hypothyroidism. Clinical Endocrinology 74:631–635

www.ingramcontent.com/pod-product-compliance
Lightning Source LLC
Chambersburg PA
CBHW060600200326
41521CB00007B/623